Jimmy,
I am told th[...]
common...that I [...]
accept this story of my journey [...]
cancer. I do not believe that cancer will
overcome you nor me. I hope that this
book will encourage and strengthen you
in your fight.

"Victory over cancer:
Live as if it were true…
because it is!"

Claiming Victory Alongside You!
Valerie Willman

Dr. Valerie Willman

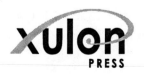

xulon
PRESS

Introduction to the Author

My name is Valerie Willman. I live on the Island of Kauai in Hawaii and have been married to Mark Willman, awesome man of God, for 21 years on June 30, 2011. Mark and I have fought some impossible battles, yet claimed the victory through our faith in Jesus Christ. The most recent battle was with breast cancer.

I was diagnosed with inter-ductal carcinoma in May of 2008. By the grace of God and the prayers of the saints, I am healed. During this amazing journey through cancer that God allowed into our lives, it became clear that he desired me to journal about my experiences.

I am astounded at how shrewdly God incorporated many miracles from my lifetime into this journal to demonstrate his love, truth and faithfulness. I believe that the Lord intends to use this writing project to communicate his encouragement and hope. I dedicate this journal to his purpose, for his glory.

A few facts that are interwoven into the journal

I have a Ph.D. in Psychology from Purdue University and a respecialization in Clinical Psychology from Illinois Institute of Technology. I have practiced as a Psychologist for 24 years. I am Board Certified as a Professional Christian Counselor by the International Board of Christian Counselors and am currently licensed in the State of Hawaii as a Clinical Psychologist.

I am a 27 time National Champion and a 5-time "Grand National/World Champion" in the sport of Baton Twirling.

I am Purdue University's 13th "Golden Girl" (Head Majorette of the All American Marching Band, and representative of Purdue University from 1983-1987).

My husband and I were separated for 2 and ½ years of our 21 year marriage and by God's divine intervention, our marriage was restored in 1996.

In the past 7 years since moving to Kauai I have claimed victory through the grace and mercy of God over: a spinal cord injury, an angioplasty of the iliac artery, and a diagnosis of two types of breast cancer.

Evidence of God's miraculous healings is demonstrated in the U-Tube Link:

http://il.youtube.com/user/valwillman

(Valerie Willman worships by twirling one, two and three batons at the "Mayor's Prayer Luncheon," "Pastor Appreciation Day," and "Church on the Beach," an outreach to the Kauai community by Kauai Bible Church.)

"Victory Over cancer" *Page Numbers*

Introduction..*vii*

<u>Journal Entries</u>
  1. Different but the same.............................17
  2. Crap sack resistance.............................18
  3. D-day.............................21
  4. God is still in control.............................22
  5. Bidden or unbidden God is present...............23
  6. Pillow story.............................24
  7. God reality.............................26
  8. Remember me.............................31
  9. Port yanking.............................34
  10. Resistance.............................36
  11. Christmas testimony.............................37
  12. Friday Fragment.............................39
  13. June already!.............................42
  14. A good name.............................42
  15. Volunteering for Relay.............................43
  16. Relay for life story.............................44
  17. Easter testimony.............................51
  18. Indy 500 and the "Miss America Dream"...........59
  19. Friends.............................64
  20. Family.............................65

21. In pursuit of the dream 71
22. Learning about the AAMB 75
23. Preparation for try-outs 78
24. And Purdue's 13th Golden Girl is… 80
25. Indianapolis 500, 2009: Our Victory March 84
26. 19th Wedding Anniversary 87
27. God numbers the hairs on our head 88
28. Registration, sleeping arrangements and
    parade security 89
29. The Golden Girls of Purdue University 91
30. Practice 95
31. Jay and Carolyn Gephart 97
32. Night before the parade 99
33. The Victory March 100
34. Race Day 103
35. First e-mail to Victory over cancer list 105
36. Initial reactions 110
37. Family and other reactions 113
38. Home group 116
39. Client reactions 117
40. The Dr. Lam experience 119
41. East vs. West 122
42. Battle with fear 123
43. Mark Willman 125
44. First surgery 128
45. Victory over cancer fight continues 132
46. The Healing 137
47. Second surgery decisions 139
48. Surgery two 141
49. Surgical success; Lymphedema fears 143
50. Second pathology report; the three 148
51. Continued treatment process 150
52. LIVE**STRONG** Manifesto 152
53. Bone scan 153
54. Annelise's heart through hair 155

55. Question 156
56. Help from Dr. Sue; Once a Month Church 158
57. More great news...161
58. ACS Volunteer visits.....................................164
59. CT and EKG 165
60. Arm rehab-Scans complete 165
61. Dr. Yee is for me! 167
62. April; a person of hope 168
63. E-mail update 169
64. Lanai anniversary trip 172
65. Emma 175
66. Researching treatments 177
67. Baton rehabilitation......................................178
68. Ukulele class 180
69. Nosode treatments..182
70. Go To The Nearest Emergency Medical Clinic ...184
71. More survival points 186
72. Oahu doctor checkups....................................187
73. Puerto Rico trip...189
74. Port flush 193
75. Oncotype results..194
76. Do you believe in miracles? Yes!......................196
77. Embodiment of the miracle..............................199
78. 9/11...200
79. Jeanne..203
80. Jeanne's miracle 206
81. Divine appointment.......................................207
82. You are what owns you 208
83. The Jeanne prayer 209
84. A final message from God................................211

Timeline of major events

4/28/08	Biopsy of tumor
5/3/08	Relay for life
5/5/08	Phone call: diagnosis cancer
5/6/08	Dr. Williams medical appointment, surgery scheduled
5/16/08	Initial Dr. Lam medical appointment and testing
5/18/08	Once-a-Month Church at Haleiwa Park on Oahu
5/20/08	Pre-op sentinel lymph node mapping
5/21/08	Surgery 1: lumpectomy with sentinel lymph node dissection
5/29/08	Pathology report from initial surgery
6/1/08-6/3/08	Kauai Bible Church fast and prayer with meeting 7-8pm at Church
6/1/08	Healing dance at Church prayer meeting
6/4/08	Surgery 2: Mastectomy with auxiliary lymph node removal
6/12/08	Second surgery pathology report
6/18/08	Dr. O appointment
6/19/08	Bone scan
6/20/08	Weekend of cancelled retreat
6/23/08	Visit from ACS representative
6/24/08	CT scan and Echocardiogram (morning)

6/24/08	Initial PT appointment (afternoon): traditional arm rehabilitation Rx
6/26/08	Second PT appointment: twirling for arm rehabilitation Rx
6/27/08	Dr. Lam medical appointment (morning)
6/27/08	Dr. Yee medical appointment (afternoon)
6/29/08	Once-a-Month Church at Haleiwa Park
6/29/08-7/6/08	Lanai Anniversary trip
7/08	Researching treatments, twirling for arm rehabilitation and Mark injecting nosodes
7/16/08	First port flush
7/25/08	First entry in Journal
7/30/08	Dr. Checkups on Oahu
8/1-8/8/08	Puerto Rico trip
8/9/08	Lost back pillow during trip to Oregon (8/9-8/18/08)
8/20/08	Second port flush
8/29/08	Doctors day on Oahu: Oncotype tumor test results; No chemo!
9/2/08	E-mail; "Do you believe in miracles… YES!"
9/11/08	Port removed
9/15/08	"Look good feel better" ACS program
10/24/08	Twirling Worship: Kauai Christian Fellowship women's Bible study
10/26/08	Twirling Worship: Pastor Appreciation Day at Kauai Bible Church
11/8/08	Kauai Women of Faith conference
11/26/08	Doctor appointments on Oahu: Checkups
12/6/08	Kauai Bible Church women's Christmas luncheon
2/20/09	Doctor checkups on Oahu
3/6/09	Vallee L. Willman's memorial service in St. Louis

3/7/09	Willman family post memorial dinner in St. Louis
4/12/09	Easter resurrection testimony: Mark and Val
4/14/09	Relay for life volunteering at ACS office
5/2/09	Relay for life at Hanapepe Stadium: twirl and testimony
5/15/09	Doctor checkups on Oahu
5/19/09	Leave for Indianapolis 500
5/22/09	Parade practice in Indianapolis
5/23/09	Indy 500 Parade: Victory March!
5/24/09	The Indianapolis 500 Race: Parade on the racetrack
6/30/09	Mark and Val's 19th wedding anniversary
8/17/09	Carolyn Gephart dies; Jay Gephart's tribute via e-mail
8/21/09	Dr. Yee checkup on Oahu
9/9/09	Dinner with Jeanne and family
9/15/09	Jeanne's call with cancer diagnosis
9/16/09	Phone call from Tennessee: prayer for Jeanne's healing
11/25/09	Call from Jeanne claiming her healing
10/21/09	Journal completed: Shirley Ayon, preliminary editor, performs her magic
4/27/11	Editing completed thanks to professional editor, Dr. Bonnie Harvey

Victory Over Cancer Journal: Introduction

In the following pages I invite you into my personal journey through cancer. I have chosen a journal format for the purpose of illustrating my daily experience. As you read my journal entries, I pray that the Lord will lead and guide you to receive the message he has especially for you.

Some of the entries will be short and others quite lengthy. You will notice significant gaps, easily identified by the dates, representing the depth of my resistance to God nudging me to write. (It's not easy pouring my heart out onto pages that I recognize will become public.) As you read you will be exposed to emotions and feelings that I wrestled with while giving God license to use my experiences as a vehicle for sharing real events, real fears and most importantly, for communicating real hope.

Whether it is you, or someone you know, in this day and age we are all affected by cancer. I pray that something I share in this book will assist you in your cancer journey.

How will you proceed? Will you give God permission to reveal his indescribable mysteries of grace and truth? Will you relinquish control over your journey through cancer to him, effectively potentiating his purpose for you within the context of impending death? Jesus, the son of God, ultimately rose from the grave and was glorified. But this happened only after he surrendered to the cross, a death of mortifying proportions, and trusted his father's plan for his life. What glory will God bring into your life and the lives of those around you, consequent of your choice to trust him and his plan for your life?

Your attitudes, your decisions *will* have an impact on others. I view it as a significant "ripple effect" in the pond of relationships. One decision, one attitude, impacts the water of the pond, sending waves of subsequent influence. Sometimes, the waves reach further than your eye can see.

I am attempting to make waves by writing this journal.

Journal Entries

Entry 1
Different but the same

I have always been told that I was "different." I liked to think of myself as a "star" shape that refused to fit into the customary "round" mold. In grade school my mother made me a skirt and vest from a zebra printed bed-spread. I wore it in conjunction with some white, knee high "go-go boots," just daring people to point me out. I pranced around tossing my head back and pointing my nose to the ceiling where I could no longer see the condemning fingers. I told myself, "I don't want to be the same as everyone else!"

I always wanted to be first: First across the finish line, first to say the answer in school, and first to forge a new way. Just leading the way wasn't good enough. Consistent with the theme of my beloved Star Trek television series, I desired; "To go where no "man" has gone before!"

I have always been told that I was "different." It has been a source of pride for me throughout my life.

Now that I have the dreaded diagnosis of cancer, I am beginning to see how very much I am the same as anyone else.

If this journal can help you navigate the extraordinary flames of chaos that cancer ignites in your life, then I believe God's purpose for me writing it will be fulfilled.

The Diagnosis

Ironically, my diagnosis day was two days after my husband, Mark, and I participated in the annual, "Relay for Life," a fundraiser sponsored by the American Cancer Society. I recall fleeting thoughts of hearing the foreboding news and how it might be to participate as one of the "Survivors." But those thoughts were pacified by the words of the medical professional who took my biopsy sample; "I will be *very* surprised if this turns out to be anything but a benign tumor." I had shared this comment with Mark, my parents, my sister and her family, my recovery Bible study group and our pastors from Kauai Bible Church. These were the only people who I had let into my potential nightmare at that time.

In my case, I really knew in my heart of hearts that the news was going to be positive...for cancer that is. If I knew then what I know now about the unfathomable transformation of life that was about to occur, and the supernatural blessings that awaited me, maybe it would have been a little easier...and maybe not. Now I am recognizing that there are just some emotional processes that are not optional in life including the amazing myriad of thoughts, feelings and behaviors that accompany the cancer journey.

Entry 2
Crap sack resistance

I just got off the phone with my sister, June, and her husband, Darryl. It's interesting how God is orchestrating this journal. I told my relatives I had begun to write yesterday, and that it has already impacted me dramatically.

I shared with them that for the past couple of months, I have been pouring over the research and current trends in cancer treatment. I must've read hundreds of articles from many sources including academic institutions, government agencies and other less "reputable" websites. Excited about what I was uncovering yesterday, I attempted to share my most recent revelations with Mark. He responded with less enthusiasm then I hoped for, saying, "That's nice, honey," promptly leaving the room for more interesting outside chores.

Aside from getting my feelings hurt, I took this to God and was impressed with the question, "aren't you spending an awful lot of time performing this research?" Well, yes I supposed I was. It then dawned on me that if I continued immersing myself in this intellectual appeasement, it would fast become an obsession.

So now what, God?

"The journal, Val, the journal."

Funny how I can instruct clients to journal their feelings and experiences, knowing full well that it will help them to process repressed, dissociated or denied emotions, but forget how important it may be for me. My brother-in-law, Darryl told me he prayed I would get this self-revelation, just in case I needed it. Well, evidently I needed it!

Yesterday I attempted to read the first page to Mark, but couldn't make it through without losing it. "What is *this*?" I thought to myself as my vocal chords began to tighten, my heart twinged with a nasty pain, and water began to fill my eyes. I thought that I was doing a great job of handling myself in this experience, thank you very much. After all, I *am* a Christian Psychologist. Not only do I have the Lord to help me move through this trial, but I have psychological training and experience helping others to identify and move through their pain. Oh my gosh! Look what's in my, "crap sack!"

Allow me to explain "crap sack," a term that my clients and co-workers are familiar with. It originated within a past counseling session where my client listened to my reflection of her tendency to stuff her, "crap" and drag it along life with her. She acted out the process, imagining herself stuffing her bad experiences and feelings into a sack; then she grasped the top, and slung it over her shoulder and began singing, "my crap-sack on my back," to the tune of Valderi Valdera, (the Happy Wanderer Song).

The "crap sack" has been one of my favorite illustrations ever since. It's such a clear picture of how we tend to carry with us the devastations of our past. Some sacks are heavier than others. Filled with massive amounts of emotional pain, the sacks inhibit our progress in life. They prevent upright relationships and they destroy our ability to receive all God has for us.

Writing this journal is one way that I am liberating myself from my cancer crap sack. I had many people suggest writing down my experiences. One such suggestion came from a co-leader in a Christ-centered 12 step program that I participate in at Kalaheo Missionary Church. Shirley Ayon has walked with me in this journey, receiving my emails and praying every step of the way. She mentioned more than once that she believed I ought to write about my experiences. Shirley teaches English at Waimea High School and is an author herself.

"Lidi" White is another lady in my Bible Study group who encouraged me, praying and strengthening me throughout my cancer journey. She has taught creative writing at the University of Hawaii extension here on Kauai. It's interesting how God placed these two women into my path, both experienced in writing, and both, prodding me to *write*!!

There were many others who shared similar encouragement, urging me to write. Sometimes God speaks quite clearly through his people.

Entry 3
D-day

"D-day" took on a new meaning for me on May 5, 2008 at about 8:30am. That was "Diagnosis day." That was when Dr. Emilia Dauway-Williams called to let me know that the biopsy sample submitted Monday, April 28th had been analyzed, and the results indicated that I had, "Inter-ductal carcinoma, the most treatable form of cancer." My mind raced as I futilely attempted to process those words...cancer... most treatable...didn't she mean, *curable*? What do we do now? What am I supposed to do? How am I going to break the news to everyone? My poor husband...oh no, my parents! What about my sister? Our church, friends, family, *clients*!!!? How am I going to break that news to all the precious ones that God sent into my office to get help from *me*?!

It was all too much. My brain was on emotion overload and I immediately went into a protective cocoon of denial and disassociation. I refused to let myself fully assimilate this death label of cancer that had just been imposed upon me. My hand continued to hold the phone but my consciousness withdrew from the immediate danger.

From what seemed to be very far away, I heard Dr. Emilia's voice saying that she would like to see me and my husband tomorrow afternoon in her office. At that time she would have a lot of information for me, and we would discuss my health situation. "Of course we will be there," I heard myself say. I was surprised at how distant and hollow the tone of my voice sounded. *Come on*, Val, you certainly are not the only one getting this type of news in your lifetime! Buck-up, pal! (Oh boy, that reminds me of one of my clients scheduled to see me today. She always calls me, "my pal, Val." How will I handle this news in my counseling sessions?)

As soon as I hung up the phone, I prayed for guidance. "Lord, help me to explain this to Mark." I dialed his number. I shared the news with him, telling him exactly what Dr. Emilia had said. There was a brief pause. He then said, "I am sorry, Val." I apologized to him as well, quite unaware of the profundity of emotional, physical and spiritual debt that I was about to incur as he unhesitatingly took on the role of "care-giver." We cried, we reaffirmed our love for one another, and we turned to the Lord with our woundedness.

Entry 4
God is still in control

Cancer wounds you. It also wounds those around you. It is hidden in the depths of your body and as such, it insidiously affects your functioning. It also affects your mind. It transforms the view you have of life itself. At the core of your being, you *will* think differently. It affects your emotions…throwing them into a chaos that relentlessly wars against you. And finally, it affects your spirit…and that is where *hope* can enter into what appears to be an impossible situation.

In that moment, my dear husband led me in claiming the truth about my diagnosis. *God is still in control.* We had many options at that defining moment. We could have stayed in the sadness, the pain, the wound…inviting bitterness and anger to brew. We could have turned immediately to God and shouted, "Why us?" (There would be a time for this and a purpose from the heart of God…but not at this particular moment.) I suppose that we also could have abandoned our faith, drawing the conclusion that this God, who is supposed to be *all* powerful and *all* merciful, had just dealt us a severe injustice. And if he is who he says he is this would never have happened. Oh thank heaven we did not choose that direction! What unfathomable blessing we would have missed!

It was our choice to claim the truth over my health. God allowed this in my life for a purpose...*his*. He would be using even this cancer experience for my good and for his glory. (*Romans 8:28,* "And we know that in all things God works for the good of those who love him, who have been called according to his purpose.")

Entry 5
Bidden or unbidden, God is present

I was awakened this morning by the Lord placing this phrase on my heart:

"Bidden or not God is present." (Phrase popularized by Carl Jung, Swiss Psychiatrist, originally attributed to Desiderius Erasmus, a Dutch humanist and theologian.)

Dr. Dan Dye, a gifted psychiatrist who I had the privilege of working with while we lived in Richland, Washington, had a phrase posted over his clinical office door. This is the translation; "Bidden or unbidden, God is present." Dan had it posted in the original Latin. Interesting, the message it conveyed via his *not* translating it into English was an even more powerful illustration of the point it made. Whether we allow ourselves to recognize the truth or not, it is still the truth. Whether we invite God into a situation, or not, he is still there.

Isn't faith related intimately to belief in the unseen? That's what *Hebrews 11:1, NKJV* tells us, "Now faith is the substance of things hoped for, the evidence of things not seen."

Entry 6
Pillow story

I am looking back to when God originally put the phrase, "Bidden or unbidden, God is present," onto my heart. It is about a month later, and finally, I am ready to record what the Lord used this for in my life.

I attempted to write while Mark and I were on a business trip to Puerto Rico but I really didn't get far. I believe that God had so much more to teach me about my diagnosis, including things that just hadn't as yet transpired. Now, as I am getting back into the swing of life here in Kauai, he is prompting me to revisit this revelation.

Here is a section from an e-mail that I sent out upon returning from our three-week trip to Puerto Rico and Oregon:

Something else we want to share with you. When we were taking our seats on the airplane from Puerto Rico to Oregon, Val realized that she had forgotten her "pillow" on the car ride to the airport. Those of you who know about Val's accident about 3 and 1/2 years ago (when her neck lost stability for an instant - much like a whiplash event - while twirling batons for the "Great Kauai Weigh-out" at the local mall) know that since that time, Val carried this pillow with her wherever she goes. There has not been a time when she traveled anywhere, or sat anytime, without it or at least some back support. The doctors who worked with Val (we lost count at 11), told her this would be something she would have to adjust to for the rest of her life. It seems that pillow became the "savior" for Val in her neck and back trauma, as it helped control the pain. We knew that someday, it would be inevitable, that the poor old thing would either be lost or just fall apart...what we did not know, is how dramatically it would affect Val.

As the realization of what was happening set in, Val began to lose it! She had visions of the past 3 and 1/2 years spinning in her head. She felt the loss of this "savior" that she had relied on for comfort and support. Then the recognition that airline travel had been the most difficult of any sitting over the years, and that now, on this International flight, she would be left without it. Also, she thought of how her parents loved to take her and Mark on long car rides over the "roller coaster like" roads of the Oregon Coast. Those swirvey, windey roads always took a toll on her neck and back, but the pillow was a great help. As the tears rolled off Val's face, Mark dove for his phone, and called the Limo Company, arranging for the pillow to be sent back to Kauai...but Val knew, the rest of the trip would be without it.

Then something that God had been working on with Val came into her mind..."Bidden or unbidden, God is present." (We originally saw this printed in Latin on a sign that was hanging over Dr. Dan Dye's office in Richland, WA. Val had worked with Dan during the time we spent in Richland before coming to Kauai.) She began to pray, saying, "It's now just you, God. I have no options here, and I bid you come forth and help me now."

*It's very interesting how God works. Val would have never given up that pillow willingly. Had this never happened, she would not have experienced the healing that God had for her...of her neck and back pain. There was no strange feeling, no warm sensation like we have heard of, but what transpired demonstrated that the promise given at the beginning of this spinal cord injury, was fulfilled. The promise was, "No weapon formed against you will prosper" (**Isaiah 54:17**).*

*Val has not experienced the pain in her neck and back as she had for the past three and one half years. She has not used any substitute "saviors" and has been able to lean back and relax in chairs, where this was proclaimed by her doctors to be impossible! We know that "With God, all things are possible" (**Matthew 19:26**). It seems Val needed to remember who her true savior was, and rely on him and him alone. We are claiming this as another miracle healing in Val's life, only by God's grace and mercy.*

We hope that all of you are doing great! We continue praying that you receive DOUBLE PORTIONS of the Blessings that you are providing in our lives. As they say here in Kauai, "Mahalo Nui Loa...thank- you very much!"

We love you all,
* Val and Mark *

Entry 7
God reality

I realize that there are many things I have not shared about myself yet in this journal, but this seemed to be something pressing and related to the cancer journey. As I pondered how God used this truth about his omnipresence to offer hope and healing in this desperate situation related to neck and back pain, I began once again to connect the dots back to a month ago, when God initially brought this to my attention.

This is what I believe. Based on my personal experience, it has given me a template for understanding myself and other diseased, struggling people. It has additionally revealed to me more of the complexity and wonder of God.

God made us in his image: *Genesis 1:27,* "So God created mankind in his own image, in the image of God he created them; male and female he created them." Within our very substance, we are made in God's image. It doesn't make any sense to me that God, who is perfect, and who told us throughout the Bible that he made us in his image, would give us imperfections. The original man and woman received everything they needed to succeed in the world that he created.

As the Bible tells us, God also gave them a choice: free will. This allowed them to decide whether or not they would obey God. We have all heard the story of how they allowed themselves to be deceived by the serpent, and in their disobedience, they invited sin into the world. As sin developed and became part of our world, everyone was and is affected by it. But how does this all relate to cancer and my journey?

I believe that God is explaining to me that cancer is a result of sin. All good comes from God. All bad comes from Satan. It really *is* as simple as that. Disease was only introduced into the world after disobedience occurred, and sin was allowed a foothold.

In case nobody has ever dared say this to you before, Satan, the evil angel that was cast out of heaven and given control over this earth, is ultimately responsible for all evil and the sin of this world, (*1 John 5:19,* "We know that we are children of God, and that the whole world is under the control of the evil one."). Satan is the author of disease, of injury, of pain and sadness. His desire is to steal, kill and destroy, (*John 10:10,* "The thief comes only to steal and kill and destroy"). It would be wonderful if we would just abolish him from this earth.

The problem is that we are also warned that Satan is extremely powerful and deceptive. He has pulled swift ones since the beginning when he tempted Eve in the Garden of Eden. As generations of people have been exposed to destructive influences of the evil one, can you imagine the genetic changes that have been compounded over the years?

Indisputably, there have been vast deteriorations from original perfection intended by our creator.

Let me attempt to provide an illustration. If I decide that I want my hair to be blonder, I can go to the beauty salon and have bleach applied to my hair. (Something I have personal experience with.) A brief exposure to bleach will lighten my hair. If bleach is applied again to my hair, most likely it will begin to fall out. As more and more bleach is applied to my head, eventually I will be bald. (Thankfully, I have not experienced this!)

If I continue applying bleach, it will begin breaking down the skin on my head. It will ultimately eat right through my skull into my brain, changing everything about me. It will even affect my personality, as it slowly destroys my ability to think, feel and process information. This may be a gruesome example, but I decided it may just contain enough power to illuminate this concept. Exposure to sin throughout thousands of years "bleaches" us with its deteriorative effects. We truly are not in the condition that our creator designed us to be.

The good news is that God is omnipotent and Satan is not. Those who decide to become children of God by asking Jesus into their hearts have access to that power. I have access to it and so do you. We do not have to stand for Satan's destruction of our bodies or minds or spirits. We have to live here on earth where we are exposed to the sin of today as well as all sin accumulated and compounded by generations past, but we are not defenseless. Far from it! We can use the power that God has given us to fight back when sin affects us. Jesus said in *Luke 10:19*, "I have given you authority to trample on snakes and scorpions and to overcome all the power of the enemy; nothing will harm you."

I do not think it coincidental that as this pillow event was unfolding in my life, I was reading a book that Jim and Katie Cassel, fellow marriage home group attendees, gave to me. The book is called, "Divine Healing: God's recipe for life and health," by Norvel Hayes. Mr. Hayes' teachings illustrate this idea from a biblical, straight forward and interestingly simple perspective.

Norvel Hayes essentially promotes the idea that God is who he says he is, and he can do exactly what he says he can do. Not only that, but he *will* do it for you-and for me! He *is* the all-powerful living God who heals. He *is* the same yesterday, today and forever. The same power that raised Jesus from the dead, that brought Lazarus back to life, that healed the blind man and stopped the bleeding for the clamoring woman, is available to us today. We just don't know how to access it. I think we get in our own way. Let me illustrate by sharing what happened to me.

When I first was injured, I could not move my neck. I had 24/7 pain. I did not know if the pain would ever cease, and neither did my doctors. It was a frightening time. I thought I was pretty good at pain management, for myself and in working with clients, until I experienced the injury. When I discovered that a pillow would lessen my persistent, excruciating pain, I was extremely grateful. I began bragging about my pillow and how it worked for me. I had my physical therapist convinced that I had the best pillow in the universe. I even went on-line to see if I could get more of this type of pillow, so all his clients could use them and feel relief as I did.

At first there was much praying and believing that the Lord intended to heal me. I received a prophetic word from two ladies at Kauai Bible Church, (Diane Beeksma and Kathy Pierson). Both ladies let me know that God wanted me to claim the scripture, "No weapon formed against you will prosper" (*Isaiah 54:17*). But as the months went by, words were spoken over me such as, "You will need to drag around that pillow the rest of your life," and "You will never be able to sit back and relax in a lounge chair like a normal person." I believed it and acted upon it. I really should not be surprised that I also gleaned the "benefits" of this defeatist "reality" that I allowed to be created in my mind.

I just have to share a story illustrating the power of this "personal reality." The main characters: my dad and I, the setting: Bandon, Oregon Community Golf Course. I still recall standing at the "tee," waiting for my turn to swing my club. This particular "par four" was a doozey. You could not see the flag designating where we were trying to hit our golf balls, because there were bushes on either side of us. As my dad walked up to take his swing, he spoke with disgust of his experience at this hole. He said that *every* time he tried to hit the ball off this "tee," he hit it directly into the nearest bush. Yes, he stated, *every time*!! Then he positioned himself over the ball, took a good, solid swing…and hit the ball into that darn bush!

I could not help myself. I laughed out loud. He turned to face me and demanded to know just *what* was so funny? I proceeded to tell him that he had just successfully predicted exactly what would happen. He knew where the ball was going, and sure enough, it went-right into that bush! He is a very smart man, and as he thought this through, he recognized that I was saying he had created the reality, and fulfilled it, just as he had imagined and believed it would be. He first created it mentally, that provoked emotions related to historical miss-hits, and finally he acted on it physically.

Dad then placed another ball on that "tee" and swung his club mightily. This one was a beauty!

Do you get it? We *do* create our own realities and we act on them. I had acted on the "reality" that my back and neck would never heal. For three and a half years I used that pillow and acted as if God would not be able to heal my body. He didn't. But, as I progressed through my cancer journey, I learned something extraordinary about my God and his ability to heal! My whole body was affected. My whole reality was changed, and this opened the door for a truth about God, the Master Healer to enter in.

I have been healed. I claim it, I believe it, and I am currently watching the reality unfold. As one of my home group members, Lady Martin, reminded me, "reality" never changes. God created the one and only *true* reality. It's the one I choose to live in.

Entry 8
Remember me

It is six days after God performed his amazing miracle in response to our prayers for all our doctors to be in agreement. God has performed a miraculous healing in me, and I do not need chemotherapy. Unreal! From eastern non-traditional doctors to western, traditionalists, they all agree. Even though I *knew* the Lord would do it, even though I can tell you *how* he did it, (that is, what factors were involved and what physically needed to occur before it all could come together), it still amazes me and boggles my mind. It reminds me just how powerful my God is.

I cannot explain why he did this for me and not for many others. As the saying goes, "There, but for the grace of God, go I." So how come I get the grace of God…but many don't? Not true. All get the grace of God if they receive it into their lives. So how come God's grace for me means healing of cancer? I do not know the answer. What I do know is how it affects me today.

While driving home from shopping this afternoon, I heard a song on the Christian radio station. I believe it was speaking to me. It is entitled, "Remember Me," by Mark Schultz. The lyrics are beautiful. They describe how God reaches out to us, making His presence known through many venues including; the Bible, in church, during prayer, through the beauty of creation, and even in emotions such as joy and peace. The defining verse portrays God promising and imploring, *"I'll remember you...remember me."*

Wow, God! How could I *ever* forget what you've done for me? The song touched something very deep inside me. I felt sadness and the tears began dripping down my cheeks as I reflected on so many who do not know their Creator God. Then I realized there have been times in my life that I did not acknowledge him. Times when I became so busy with my life that I forgot to read out of my Bible, or I just didn't have the minute it takes to read my home page on my computer. (Mark and I pull up the "Daily Bread" on our home page, a Christian devotional by RBC Ministries.) And, I was much too busy to get onto my knees and pray. (My faithful husband, Mark, says, "It's the best way to begin and end each day...on your knees.") And the time between clients was spent recording clinical data instead of making sure to pray for the private struggle that God had just allowed me the privilege of entering into with the person. And sometimes I did not even make it to women's Bible study at Kauai Christian Fellowship on Friday because I had too much paperwork to complete and errands to run.

Lord, forgive me. Let me never be caught up into the world in this way again. It is clearer to me now more than ever before, that when I do allow myself to be swept up into this frenzied, pressured life pace, I pay for it. The effects are insidious. First I begin to feel the tightness in my muscles. Next, I may or may not realize that I am getting cranky...a state that Mark has no problem identifying.

Other effects may take the form of inefficiency. Yes, inefficiency. Weird isn't it? I have this inaccurate belief that pushing myself to go faster and faster will actually propel me forward with accelerated speed, but what it really accomplishes is prevention of smooth completion of tasks. It fosters jerky, uncoordinated efforts in whatever I am doing. The process snowballs as long as it is allowed to continue. It creates more and *more* chaos for me until I am so exhausted or in so much pain that I drop to my knees…finally. In the meantime, I have just succeeded in producing so much "chemical crap" (that's a technical term I use for harmful physiological changes), that my body is left reeling. I now realize that this cycle of actions contributes to creating an effective internal environment for growing and developing cancer cells.

I've done it for so long I cannot remember the first time that I engaged in this pressure producing manner. I know it wasn't common practice for me at five years old, when I began to take hula lessons from Lena Robertson in my home town of Richland, WA. Lena, a native of Molokai, Hawaii, was forever emphasizing the importance of *gracefulness*. With slow, definite movements commonly used in traditional Hula to tell a beautiful story, it is nothing to be rushed or pressured. My sister, June was much better at this than I was.

I do recall a time when I was about 14 years old, when our baton twirling group helped out with the concession stand at the "Miss Tri-Cities" pageant. I couldn't help thinking to myself that there were *some* of us who were very quick in getting the ice in cups, filling them with pop, and serving the customers, while others seemed to take *forever*! (Just to clear up a potential misnomer, June was one of the quickies!) Maybe what appeared to be an asset was actually a detriment.

This afternoon I was shopping and getting hungry. It really bothers me to pay for a huge plate of food, and only eat a tiny portion of it. I decided that Walmart, where I was shopping, was right next to the Wilcox Memorial Hospital, and the hospital had a nice cafeteria with a salad bar. The food is weighed, so you only pay for what you really want. I like that! Anyway, on the way in, God showed me something that I never noticed before. There, just before you enter the cafeteria, is a chapel.

I believe God desired for me to be alone with him for a few minutes, because it was just me and him. The pressure and hurriedness began melting away. I felt compelled to thank him for the gift of life that he had renewed in me. Life truly *is* a gift. Now that I am typing this out, I recall hearing that very truth on the radio prior to entering the hospital. (It was confirmation!) Life is precious, and I know now more than ever, how fragile it can be. I hope that I do not take my life for granted any more, ever again.

Entry 9
Port yanking

I just returned from getting my "port" removed. It was placed into the skin above my right breast during my second surgery, in anticipation of chemotherapy. Its purpose was to allow direct access into my veins, so that the chemicals from chemotherapy would have the best shot at killing any stray cancer cells. Since I received God's blessing of *no need for chemo*, and agreement from my oncologist, Dr. Yee, the port got yanked.

Dr. Emilia, (my breast cancer surgeon), listened to my testimony of how God pulled off the incredible miracle of getting all my doctors into agreement via the extremely low Oncotype DX Breast Cancer Assay score. She seemed pleased. I am not sure that she saw it as a miracle. But then, *who does?*

You would expect that my reaction to this procedure would be to rejoice and praise God!!! I did call my husband, who had forgotten that I had the appointment today, (as did I). I told him the port was *out*. "I'm free, I'm free...it's gone and I'm free!" was what I said. So, why do I not feel that freedom totally? How come at this moment, as I type these words, I am experiencing sadness, even pain in my chest and heart? I am uncertain.

This cancer deal is incredibly taxing emotionally, and at times like this, very confusing. Could it be that I am actually *sad* that this cancer journey is winding down? Is it pain for those diagnosed with cancer that must go through chemotherapy? Or is it just the letdown of my emotions after trudging through the past few months? At this point it is unclear to me. What I do know is that my "victory over cancer" team seems to be dwindling in the obvious support that they were providing me...at least it feels that way. The e-mails that used to come in response to an update Mark and I sent, (sometimes even before we logged off the computer), are absent. The urgency is gone, and folks seem to be taking their time in responding with rejoicing and praising God for all he has done.

At some point I wondered if there were some who just cannot believe that God really *has* healed me, and their silence is an effort to keep from making condemning remarks about our decisions against further treatment. Maybe this idea comes from my experience earlier in this process, when fingers of my western medical practitioners were pointed at my eastern medical practitioners, threatening death without traditional treatment. As has been customary in my life, taking a non-traditional, even non-conforming, route puts me at risk for this reaction from those who generally walk unobtrusively with the crowd, and prefer that you link your arms with theirs.

I believe that people do the very best they can to walk through the struggles of life with their friends and family, but we are so ill-equipped for this. Nobody teaches us in school how to support each other through inevitable trials and crises. Our parents did not learn either, so they do their best and tend to struggle with this too. As a psychologist, I recognize that it is not during the beginning of a tragedy or loss when people most need the social support, but surprisingly, it is after the music fades, and the band packs up for home, and nobody is there…that the biggest need arrives. Most likely this is due to our ineptness in dealing with our own emotions.

Sigmund Freud, the famous Swiss psychiatrist, identified human tendency to use defense mechanisms to prevent ourselves from overdosing on emotions and becoming incapacitated. I am a pretty good illustration of using minimization, dissociation and denial to get through the most demanding facets of this cancer process. Taken to the extreme, these coping techniques are unhealthy, but used in moderation, for times like these, they are necessary. When the support seemingly dissipates after the immediate, obvious needs subside, then the emotions which were suppressed, disguised and ignored, must begin to surface.

I guess I really do know that if I wanted to, I could call on people from our "victory over cancer" e-mails, or anybody in our affiliated churches, or other folks we know. I believe that any one of them would be more than happy to help me pour out my emotional crap sack…well, *most* anyone! It seems that there is something inside me that recognizes that I have asked quite enough from my faithful supporters, and that it is time that I dealt with the emotions alone, with my Lord. He is my ever-present help in time of need and the one who never has to put me on hold or coordinate schedules with me. Jesus…thank you, that you are *always* available. Thank-you, Lord, for never balking at how heavy my "crap sack" is.

Excuse me while I go and pray off this crap…

Entry 10
Resistance

There has been a gnawing at my heart to get back to typing this journal. I can't even participate in my Friday morning women's Bible study without the Lord speaking through the lessons about it. I tell you, it better be because someone will benefit from the effort...maybe *moi* (me)?!

I have a difficult time organizing things. Over the years I have had to really concentrate on learning strategies for this. Maybe what I should do is use a logical order for relating my experience in this cancer journey. I'll begin at the beginning. Write that down, will you? (That was a joke regarding my stating the obvious). Since I have already started to tell you about the initial shock of being diagnosed with cancer, I will continue from where I left off.

Entry 11
Christmas testimony

About two months have passed since I last wrote in this journal. It's interesting how God has attempted to get my attention redirected back to this journal, but I have not been cooperating. I almost feel like one of those "bobble head dolls" as I have nodded over and over, sure Lord, uh-huh, yes, I will get right on it! But then the dirty laundry seemed so alluring, and then there was ironing, and of course, answering e-mails, and piddling around with whatever life was bringing over the past month. It took a bit of pride-bashing for him to accomplish the task.

This past week Kauai Bible Church held the annual women's Christmas party. I realized about three days ahead of time that I had not signed up or paid. (Oh my, I *still* haven't paid). Moving right along... I called the office to make sure I was welcome, only to discover that my testimony was being counted on for the program! I love to share what the Lord has done for me, so this was OK with me. However, it meant putting something together quickly, because I had also inherited the responsibility for teaching the women's Sunday school because our fearless leader and Pastor's wife, Darlene had contacted a contagious illness.

I proceeded to pray and what do you know?! God had me print out this journal and read it over, looking for appropriate illustrations for my testimony. I noticed that there were significant gaps in my writings. In fact, I had only just begun to really tell my story. There was so much more I desired to share. *Wow*, I hadn't even written about that or *that*!! Good grief, I said to myself, I really need to get going on this again!

And then…the women's Christmas party came and went without a peep from me! Can you imagine that?! I was *not* asked to share my testimony. It was a fabulous evening of fellowship, food and love. Many guests of the Kauai Bible women were touched deeply and we all applauded our incredible hostess, Diane Beeksma, for her giftedness in hospitality and talents of creative design and décor. The Christmas Spirit abounded and it was a *huge* success…all without *my testimony*!!! So, what is this about, God?

The journal, Val. The journal.

There is something else too. When I received the news that I did not have to go through chemotherapy, I realized that I would be able to get back into counseling again. At that time, there was a significant question in my mind regarding how quickly I should pick up my client load. After prayer and discussion with Mark, I decided to let God make the decision. I prayed and re-dedicated my clinical practice to the Lord, telling him that I would wait on his referrals. I knew that I could make a few calls and send a few letters, and the new clients would come rolling in, but this was not what I knew God wanted me to do. So, I waited on him.

The client calls came flooding in. In about a week I had a full load plus four on a waiting list! But, it is amazing how this played out. Some of the clients did not show up. Some of them cancelled. When I got to the point where I was able to call the folks on my waiting list, they had either gone elsewhere, or decided they did not really want counseling at that time.

I knew that God was taking care of me. The message to me was that he desires me to continue working as a psychologist, but there is something *else* that he wants my attention on. He is providing time for *something else.* What on earth could it be?

The journal, Val. The journal.

Entry 12
Friday Fragment

Bill Dean, Director of Northwest Indiana's Youth for Christ, sent me an e-mail today. A wonderful article from Dan Wolgemuth, President of Youth for Christ/USA, was included. I almost did not read it. Something...some*one* prompted me to and I am blessed because of it.

Friday Fragments: January 16, 2009

Ray Fitzgerald had the good sense to marry my wonderful niece in early 2001. The ceremony took place in the suburbs of Washington, D.C. and was a delightful celebration of love, life and hope.

Today, over eight years later, Ray and Kristin have converted promises made into promises kept. They are making good on the public commitment to care for each other in sickness and health. Today, Ray Fitzgerald fights cancer. He's been fighting it for over seven months. He's fighting with every weapon he has and can acquire. Through pain, exhaustion and uncertainty... Ray, with Kristin at his side, has raised a fist to this monster.

Cancer is a hideous disease that thrives on lies that it communicates to the very cells it lives beside. It's mutinous and cowardly. It's selfish and disgusting. There is no mercy, no respect and no limit to the evil of this hell birthed plague. We are right to want to scream out indignantly at this terror, for it arose from the lying schemes of a fallen world. It is not a creation of the garden. It was conceived after God declared His creation "good." It is part of that which will be no more in heaven.

Yet, lest we declare defeat, lest we raise the white flag prematurely... let me reflect on the lessons being taught in the classroom of Ray and Kristin. For out of this vigilante evil, God has mobilized an organized army that is learning in the war room.

There are no asterisks next to the verses in Romans 8 that declare that nothing can separate us from the love of Christ. Cancer was not ignored or overlooked when the apostle Paul proclaimed that we are more than conquerors.

Ray and Kristin are turning back this evil... not with medical prowess, but with faith and tenderness and vulner-ability and visibility. They have answered the call by ele-vating the fight. They have not eradicated the disease, they are redeeming it... even as they remain in the fight.

Ajith Fernando writes... "Suffering brings the real issues of life to the surface. In the midst of suffering you see whether what a person has lived for has served him or her well" (The Call to Joy and Pain).

And so, as one of the mobilized throng, I commend Ray and Kristin... who have emboldened me to fight well against the lying, destructive schemes of the evil one. And in the war room, I find my heart and soul stirred to fight against all of the evil strategies of our foe. For every injustice, every selfish act, every hopeless lie finds its match and more in the death defying life of Jesus.

Ray and Kristin... I love you, honor you... and stand ready to fight... with you, for you, because of you.

Dan Wolgemuth
(Reprinted with permission)

There are two points that Dan Wolgemuth makes that touched me most profoundly. The first is his description of cancer:

"Cancer is a hideous disease that thrives on lies that it communicates to the very cells it lives beside. It's mutinous and cowardly. It's selfish and disgusting. There is no mercy, no respect and no limit to the evil of this hell birthed plague. We are right to want to scream out indignantly at this terror, for it arose from the lying schemes of a fallen world. It is not a creation of the garden. It was conceived after God declared His creation "good." It is part of that which will be no more in heaven."

For me, this is validating to read. The powerful truth that cancer was never meant to be, that God did not originally intend us to be exposed to this parasitical monster, equips me with increased resolve to defend myself against it. The fact that cancer has to resort to lying in order to exist clearly demonstrates its relationship to the evil one.

Dan goes on to say:

"There are no asterisks next to the verses in Romans 8 that declare that nothing can separate us from the love of Christ. Cancer was not ignored or overlooked when the apostle Paul proclaimed that we are more than conquerors."

I love that. No asterisks. There are *no* exceptions. Cancer cannot take us from the omnipotent love of Jesus. I am claiming *Romans 8:28*, "And we know that in all things God works for the good of those who love him, who have been called according to his purpose."...*no asterisk*!!! In *all things*, God wins! He takes the devil's efforts to kill, steal and destroy, and he converts them into good; my good. That's awesome. That's empowering.

Entry 13
June already!

How could it possibly be *June* already?! I have succeeded in ignoring the Lord's prompting to continue this
journal for six months. In response, he has cleared my plate
of everything else that has been taking my time, including
counseling. Amazing how he did that. During the beginning
of the year I had plenty of referrals, and old clients checking
in, but I am down to pretty much nothing...zero...ziltcho!
OK, Lord, I hear you, and this time, I plan to obey.

Entry 14
A good name

We just returned from a trip to the mainland for my
father-in-law's funeral. Vallee L. Willman had been in a
nursing home for over two years, and God determined his
purpose here with us was finally completed. We rejoiced in a
"life well lived." Dr. Vallee L. Willman spent his life serving
people using his talents to become a very famous heart surgeon, heading up the Department of Surgery at St. Louis
University. His faithful wife of 57 years, Melba Willman,
raised their nine children. She also managed to contribute
to the university hospital with creative programs that even
today continue to influence the way patients and families are
cared for. As I prayed for the Lord to give me a Scripture
to share with the Willman family, my tiny little travel Bible
opened to this Scripture:

Proverbs 22:1, "A good name is more desirable than great
riches; to be esteemed is better than silver or gold."

Dr. Vallee L. and Melba Willman cultivated a "good name" and we continue to reap the benefits of their dutiful faith and service-filled walk on this earth.

Entry 15
Volunteering for Relay

The most recent development in my journey through cancer came from an unexpected source. I knew that "Relay for Life," the American Cancer Association's annual fund raising event in Hanapepe Stadium, was coming up very soon. I had been prompted in my heart to visit the ACS office and volunteer to help. As usual, I had waited until the last minute to follow through.

I entered the office, and was connected with the lady who was organizing the program for Relay. We bantered about many potential directions for my contribution, when finally, I said, "I think I need to tell you something." The Lord had directed me to expose my motive for volunteering. I proceeded to describe to her what the Lord had allowed me to experience over the past year, and made it perfectly clear that my goal was to *tell* people about the Lord's faithfulness to me, give examples of the role he played in my healing, and offer a demonstration of the miraculous healing by twirling my batons. I said, "If this is too much Jesus for you, just tell me. I won't be offended." This caught her off guard, but her response masterfully portrayed God's handiwork and orchestration of the intangibles necessary to pull it off in this day and age. She said, "Well, I am also a Christian. Your timing is perfect, because I have a meeting tonight with the directors, and I can run this by them and let you know tomorrow."

Wow!! I already knew the answer before her e-mail the next day confirmed it. Mark and I would be allowed to give our testimony, and I was invited to twirl both regular and fire-batons. (We decided the fire twirling would be perfect for the later evening performance times when it would be dark out.) My choice of song was approved, giving me the go-ahead on the theme: "When I call on Jesus," by Nicole C. Mullen, from *Philippians 4:13, NKJV,* "I can do all things through Christ who strengthens me." *How perfect!!*

My efforts through those ensuing ten days were directed towards writing out the cancer journey, memorizing each line, and practicing both the delivery and my baton twirling routine. I began practicing my "speech" in our dining room, in front of our ever-so-attentive cat, Pumpkin, and progressed to announcing my testimony to the entire valley below the Hanapepe Canyon lookout at the side of the highway. (*That* was an inspiration from God. Prompted by my fondness for this beautiful roadside attraction, I recited my lines while tourists kept their distance from this strange woman who was speaking with obvious passion and conviction... to herself!)

And then, Saturday came. By that time, Mark and I had practiced several times together. He had prepared an introduction that included recognition of the Pioneer Seed Company's Relay team, who had raised amazing amounts of financial support for the effort over the past seven years. In fact, Pioneer Seed was honored by the ACS as the top financial supporter of the year.

Entry 16
Relay for life story

It has been a couple weeks since I added anything to this journal. I can't really say why this is the case. I tell my clients that they are experiencing "resistance" when they have a difficult time addressing something they really need to do. Strong emotions interwoven into the issue snag the therapeutic process. It is akin to avoidance. I don't know if this is what I am experiencing or not.

At any rate, I believe that I would like to be used as a vehicle for God's message of hope and possibilities, and this journal may be a way to convey this message. Truly, I have *much* to say.

"Relay for Life"

The American Cancer Society organizes a fund raiser each year called, "Relay for Life." I have mentioned this previously. It was one year ago, two days after Mark and I participated in the event, when I received the cancer diagnosis. But this year was different. This year was personal.

In the three years that we participated in the Hanapepe "Relay for Life" we had always wondered what went on in the "Survivors Tent." We really didn't want to find out *this* way! It was pretty humbling to meet people who have battled cancer for many, many years, and hear their stories. I began to wonder if my testimony was even worth telling in the presence of such courageous people. (Oh yes, Satan would just love for me to believe that!)

I joined in the "Survivor victory lap" that traditionally kicks off the Relay. It was amazing walking around the track, seeing all those supporters and hearing the applause. Inside I kept reminding myself that I wanted to be able to do this again, and again, and again. It was inspirational for me. One of my doctors even took a picture of me as I passed by him! (Dr. Thomas Williamson as well as his colleague, Dr. Steven Penner, at the Kauai Medical Clinic in Eleele, played a significant role in my life since my move to Kauai, especially since the cancer diagnosis. They truly are two of my "heroes.")

Mark joined with me, as my "care-giver," for the traditional second lap of the Relay. We waved and joked as we went around, but there was a significant element of nostalgic heaviness settling into our minds and hearts. It is so amazing how many, many people are affected by this disease, and how strong the support seems to be for one another.

As the night wore on, we began preparing for our testimony. Because we live just up the hill from the track, we went home to change, and to rehearse one more time. Too bad! As I attempted to recite my lines, I got stuck right near the beginning. How irritating! Mark assured me that it would not happen when the "lights went on me," but I am pretty sure I was not consoled.

We returned to the track and waited our turn. Then it came...and I got stuck. It was the kind of stuck that notes would do nothing for. I was completely lost. I paced back and forth a couple times, praying for guidance, saying something stupid in a feeble attempt to jolt my mind. I can explain this "brain fart" by putting on my psychologist's hat and recognizing the intensity of emotions I was attempting to manage. Mark says it was not that bad...I am just describing how it felt to me. After what seemed to me like an eternity had passed, God helped me to get back on track. Here is the transcript in its entirety:

Transcript of Val's cancer Journey: "Relay for Life," Hanapepe, HI May 2, 2009

Thank-you so much for this opportunity to share our cancer journey with you.

On the Monday following last year's "Relay for Life," I received the diagnosis of "breast cancer." I would never wish this experience on anyone. What a shock! I cannot begin to describe the overwhelming feelings of disbelief, of fear and of helplessness that I experienced...however, I would never change it. The diagnosis has been an unbelievable blessing in my life. I have experienced a deeper level of love, faithfulness and power of God that I would not have been capable of gaining any other way. Additionally, I discovered something that, for me, only existed previously in the Scriptures. It is the "peace that surpasses all understanding." The Bible told me that there was such a thing, a peace not of this world, or of any situation...but completely of God. It is in this peace that I have learned to live with this cancer diagnosis.

It was shortly after my initial meeting with my breast surgeon that I was scheduled for a "lumpectomy and sentinel lymph node biopsy." We also sought non-traditional medical treatment, and believe that we had divine guidance in obtaining that support.

After the surgery, results jolted us into reality, as our doctor gave us very bad news. There were not just one, but two forms of cancer present. Cell activity had increased, and it was believed that the cancer had spread into my lymphatic system. As Mark and I shared tears and an embrace in the office that day, we determined that the question was not, "Why us?" but instead, "Why not us?!" You see, we are Christians, and we believe the Lord will see us through anything, using "all things for our good and for his glory." Do we really trust the Lord unconditionally? It was clear to us that we were being called to confirm our faith in his sovereignty over our lives.

During this battle against cancer, we were given the scripture, Isaiah 54:17, NKJV, "No weapon formed against you shall prosper." We claimed that scripture, as well as many other healing scriptures alongside our church families at Kauai Bible Church, Kalaheo Missionary Church, and Kauai Christian Fellowship. We were joined by our families and Christian brothers and sisters here on Kauai, as well as many others around the world. It seemed to us that every day we were being added to another prayer list, by friends and family members here and on the mainland. I received a phone call one day from someone I did not know, who said that she had heard about my situation, and felt lead by the Lord to call and give me a confirmation of how much God loves me! Kauai Bible Church declared a three-day fast with prayer on our behalf and it was during that time between surgeries that we believe I was healed of cancer. I said that cancer did not stand a chance next to the incredible power of God through these wonderful, faithful people in my life. I underwent a second surgery to perform a mastectomy and complete lymph node resection, and this time when the results came back, they were all incredibly good news!

After giving us our great results, our surgeon gave us some sobering news. She had been required to present very sad news that same week to three women who were in similar situations. At that point we dedicated our prayer team to praying for the three, representing all those diagnosed with cancer. We wear the "LIVESTRONG" bracelets to represent the three, banding us together to fight this cancer battle, and to reinforce our commitment to pray for the three, and to "LIVESTRONG in Jesus."

We were then connected to an oncologist who promptly recommended "hard-core" chemotherapy, not just one round, but two or more, and likely radiation treatments to follow. I finally decided to call the American Cancer Society, and they ran to my aid. I was visited by a knowledgeable, supportive volunteer, who gave me encouragement and lots of information. (Thank you, Susan Campbell!) She answered my questions and suggested I attend the program, "Look good-feel better," presented at the ACS office.

It was awesome! The volunteers provided me with products, connections with other survivors, and loving assistance in learning how to bring out that image of God, to look good and feel at my best, no matter what road we chose to travel in our cancer journey.

And there were decisions to be made. All my doctors reminded me that these decisions were "life or death," but there was disagreement in the direction. There was such profound disparity in opinions that my eastern medical team stood on one end of the continuum while my western medical team stood on the opposite end. They pointed at each other saying the exact same thing, "If you do what they say to do, you will surely die." Mark and I stood in the middle of the continuum, looking up to God, praying for his wisdom and direction.

I poured myself into research, searching for the right way for us. With tremendous prayer coverage, and with the help of my dad, I discovered a new test that had yet to be commonly used in a case like mine. When I presented the information to my new oncologist, he determined that it would be appropriate for me, and he went to work coordinating efforts to perform the test. He stated, "I know you...if this test indicates a need for chemotherapy, you'll be the first in line." I thought about that. First in line? I finally responded, "Yes, I believe if that is God's will for me, I absolutely would be!"

The day he gave me my results is still fresh in my mind. I restated what my doctor had just told me, saying, "So, doctor, let me be sure I understand you...God has performed a miraculous healing in me and I do not need chemotherapy." And he replied, "Yes, God has performed a miracle, and you do not need chemotherapy." We celebrated and praised God for his mercy and healing miracle. There were "high-5's" all around the office that day!

Without the research money of the American Cancer Society, and all of you, it would not have happened. Because you were there, and you were willing, the time, support and money you gave through the ACS went to development of the tool my doctor used to determine I did not need chemotherapy treatment.

I am so very grateful to all of you for playing a part in my healing. God's work through you allows me to live today and to share with you the gifts and talents God has blessed me with. I invite you to not focus on me but on the miracle

God performed through all of you, allowing this opportunity to worship him in this way, today.

We remember the three representing all who have and will have the cancer diagnosis, and we trust God with that which we fail to understand. Join with me tonight as I praise him and remember, when you call on Jesus, all things truly are possible!

And then, I performed my Baton Twirling routine to "Call on Jesus," by Nicole C. Mullen. It seemed a bit difficult for me to focus, but as I twirled and became more comfortable on the little stage and low ceiling, the movements flowed just about as I had practiced. Then the time came in the song to make a mad dash off the back edge of the stage, and run into the loving "flames" of my dear husband, who had just lit the end of my fire baton for me! (During the 10 minutes prior to our testimony, Mark had made sure that the fire baton ends were nice and soaked with white gas, so that at the appropriate time, he could light'em up!)

As the song began to crescendo, I spun and tossed my fire baton. Before the end of the song, I ran over to Mark with my flaming baton, tossed it down and picked up two-fire batons for him to light up. As I ran back to center stage twirling the two-fire batons, Mark feverishly worked to put out the baton that I had tossed at him, just missing the towel he had neatly set out for me as the target for the drop off! As always, Mark accomplished his part of the routine, and I also completed the testimony with a "no-drop routine."

As we put out the two remaining fire batons together, people rushed up to the front of the stage. I couldn't believe my eyes! They formed a long line, and began to take turns hugging me and telling me how God had touched their hearts through our testimony. At one point I began to feel a bit embarrassed, as there was soon to be another "act" coming on stage. Thankfully, the Lord had managed to take care of that too, as the fairly large musical group took a while to set up. By that time, the line had ended and we had gathered our stuff up to leave. I was humbled by the experience. Mark and I prayed that the Lord would water any seeds that were planted in the hearts of listeners that evening.

I did wonder why the line of people formed, and I came to the conclusion that it might have partially been for the ACS to see. I had been concerned that they may have had regrets about asking us to give this blatantly Christian testimony at such a public event. I may never know what they really thought. I still have not heard a peep out of any of them about that night, at least not yet. What I do know is that I will be forever grateful to them for giving us the opportunity to tell our story of hope, and to give God the glory!

Entry 17
Easter testimony

If Relay only knew what a *miracle* it was that I was able to perform for them! Ahhh…that was included in a different testimony. Our Easter testimony!

Easter, 2009

This year Mark and I were given the honor of speaking at the Kauai Bible Church Easter Service. Each year our church pastors and tiny congregation of about 200 members, work tirelessly to put on a *huge* Easter service at a local hotel. This year, as in many years past, it was at the Kauai Hilton Resort. We attracted about 365 people this year. What a blessing!

The topic of the day was naturally, "Resurrection." Mark and I have had so many resurrections in our lives that it was a perfect assignment for us. I began by telling about my health traumas over the past four and half years, ending with the cancer diagnosis. Then I twirled, demonstrating the miraculous "resurrection" of my physical body, allowing me to perform the intricate twirling, spinning and dancing movements of a former "Grand-National/World Champion."

Mark then described the resurrection that God performed in his life, bringing him from the pit of despair, depression, and addiction, back to life abundant in Jesus! Mark's story is an amazing testimony in itself, culminating in a life-saving experience of salvation at an Indianapolis "Promise Keepers" Conference.

Then we told about our experience of God's resurrection power in our marriage. We told about our "Miracle on Molokai," and shared our faith and renewed strength as we fastened our marriage onto the "solid rock" of our Lord Jesus Christ. We never get tired of telling how God brought us both to our knees, and restored what we had destroyed.

Here is the transcript of our message:

2009 Easter Testimony Outline
I. Intro to theme of resurrection (1 min)

VAL: *Happy resurrection Sunday everybody! We are very privileged to be here today to share with you the resurrection that God has performed in our lives. Let me introduce to you my handsome, loving, God-serving husband, from St. Louis, MO, currently working as a corn breeder for Pioneer Seed in Waimea...Dr. Mark Willman.*

MARK: *This is my beautiful, pretty wife, Valerie Willman, from Richland, WA who works as a Christian Psychologist at Kaua'i Bible Church.*

When I met Val Ludwick in 1987 at Purdue University in Indiana, she was finishing her Ph.D. in Psychology and I had just completed my Ph.D. in Plant Breeding, I promised her we would move west – like Washington (where she was from) someday. Little did I know the Lord Jesus would lead us to

52

Kauai. Today, we "a pair of Docs" are going to share with you the story of our dead lives and destroyed marriage resurrected by the living God. In the literal sense of the word, resurrection refers to the event of a dead person completely returning to life: You be the judge as we share with you our stories of resurrection in our lives.

II. Resurrection of Val's life (3 min)

VAL: 4 and half years ago when we moved to Kauai, we brought with us a ministry that God had developed, using my baton twirling as a vehicle to communicate his power and glory. During one ministry opportunity at Kukui Grove mall, I was performing my routine, and my head momentarily lost its stability, and whipped back. As in many whiplash-type accidents, I didn't realize until the next day when I had the worst headache I had ever experienced, what damage had been created. The following day it was so bad I could not turn my head, and I was in pain 24 hours per day. After seeking help from over ten doctors and professionals, we still did not know whether my pain and physical condition would ever change.

Two years ago, as I was walking for exercise, my leg went dead on me. It just quit working. There was pain, so I stopped, and it resolved itself, so I continued. In the next couple of weeks this kept on happening, progressing to the point where I could not walk from my car in the parking lot, to the grocery store, without it going "dead." After two months, the problem was diagnosed as, "fibro muscular dysplasia," something the doctors knew very little about. An angioplasty was performed on my iliac artery above my leg, in hopes that it would open the circulation up and help with the problem.

And one year ago, I discovered a lump that was subsequently diagnosed as breast cancer. I underwent two surgeries and holistic treatment.

As we walked through these health challenges, we were given the scripture Isaiah 54:17, NKJV, "No weapon formed against you shall prosper, and every tongue which rises against you in judgment you shall condemn. This is the heritage of the servants of the LORD, and their righteousness is from me, says the LORD."

We claimed this scripture over each of my health problems, along with Kauai Bible Church and so many others who prayed with us and supported us, and I stand before you today claiming Victory...over the spinal cord injury...Victory over the leg injury... to this day God continues to heal me and give me greater flexibility and freedom of movement...and I claim Victory over cancer.

In the name of Jesus Christ, my Lord and Savior, and my master healer. He is the resurrector of my body, and the reason I can twirl and worship with you today!

MARK: *So now, Val will share with us in the way she worships her savior, through baton twirling. Val trained and competed for over 16 years in this sport, won many trophies, including five Grand- National/ World titles and 27 National titles. In fact, she will be part of this year's Indianapolis 500 parade and opening ceremonies this Memorial day week-end.*

Join us as Val "Celebrates Jesus".....

III. Twirling (3 min) Song: "Celebrate Jesus," by Gary Oliver, and performed by: The Alleluia Singers

III. Mark's resurrection and Marriage resurrections (13 min); Brief chronological story of Mark's bodily destruction & resurrection

> MARK: *Can you believe how God has raised this shrunken shrink?!?*
>
> *As Val cools down, let me tell you how I destroyed my life and marriage and how Christ restored me. Even though I looked successful on the outside, I was a corn breeder for a food company; I was slowly killing myself and my marriage by abusing alcohol and pursuing my fleshly desires. It wasn't until Val had enough of me and my antics that she confronted me and told me she was leaving me. It was at that time I decided to get help.*
>
> *I quickly got into recovery. Through the help of local churches, friends, and the men's organization Promise Keepers, I was able to develop a new relationship with Jesus, receive his forgiveness for my wrongs, and begin to live a new life with him, free from the alcohol addiction I had allowed in my life.*
>
> *As I developed a growing relationship with Jesus through daily prayer, Bible reading, and hanging with other Christians, His Spirit revealed to me the lust issues in my life that were interfering with living the life he had for me, even though God had taken away the obsession to drink.*
>
> *As with the booze, the All-Powerful God, lead me to people who through their help, prayers and His resurrection power, freed me from this powerful presence in my life. By the grace of God and through the fellowship of his Spirit and others, I have not found*

it necessary to drink alcohol or act-out for over 10 years. If you are struggling with issues of this kind, I am here to tell you there is hope and freedom through Jesus.

Marriage transformation chronologically

VAL: *While Mark struggled with his issues, I was battling my own addiction that contributed to our marital problems. My "drug of choice" was food. By turning to food when I felt lonely, or anxious, I was slowly isolating myself emotionally from my husband. I didn't see this, and blamed him for all our problems. I told him "you're killing yourself and I'm not gonna die with you." And, I left the marriage. In fact, I eventually left the state of Indiana where we lived, and moved to Oregon. I lived as if we were divorced, looking to food and other relationships for the answers to my pain. It was in Oregon that God began showing me the truth about my life. I began to see a Christian Psychologist to work on my eating disorder issues. God made it clear to me by the end of that year that I needed to move back to Indiana, which I did, fully expecting to file for divorce, finish my year as Assistant Professor at Purdue University North Central, and move on with my life. I'm so grateful God had other plans! I still remember the day he finally reached my heart. I was at the foot of my bed, crying out to God with the Bible open to the Psalms, saying, "I know my way leads to the pit of "H-E-double toothpicks" and I don't want to be there anymore. Please, God, take back my life. Tell me what to do." And He did. He told me to go speak with my pastors about what I had been doing for the last two years. They directed me to speak with Mark. Mark had us pray and wait. After about two weeks of praying and asking God for his direction...Mark called and asked me out on a date. We began to date...but it was horrible! We weren't getting anywhere! After a couple of months of this, Mark was assigned a trip to Molokai, Hawaii for work. He called and asked if I would accompany him, so we could continue to work on our marriage. I said yes, believing that the worst case scenario was that I would get a good vacation out if the deal! So... we went to Molokai together.*

MARK: *It turns out God had a plan for this trip. You see from my perspective, I had this work trip and I thought I could use it as a last ditch effort to spend time with Val to "save" our marriage. So I thought we would have plenty of time to connect on Moloka'i – "Eh, slow down, this is Moloka'i" right? Well, after two days, it was the same thing. I would work in the morning and we would "date" in the afternoon and evening, but still not talking about the issues that were keeping us apart. So I suggested on the third day to go to Kalaupapa lookout (overlooking the former leper colony).*

VAL: *It was hot, I was so tired and frustrated, and I prayed: "Just tell me, God. I don't care what the answer is. Just let me know if we are going to be able to put our marriage back together or not, so that I can enjoy this vacation!"*

MARK: *As we walked down the trail, we met this African American couple, Clinton and Margaret Davis. We told them we were here to fix our marriage. They told us they were here to do God's work – whatever that would be and they happen to work with couples in the church they pastor on Oahu. Clinton asked if they could work with us now. We agreed. We prayed and then started working on small and then bigger commitments between each other. Finally, when he asked me if I would be willing to have Val move back in with me, I had to say "No," not until we resolve where we were to live. You see Val wanted to move west and I was indifferent about where we go – just as long as I had a job. So we prayed and they sent us on the trail to hammer-out this issue. God's Spirit gave us the solution to this problem shortly after we sat down. How do I know it was God's Spirit? I recently heard someone say, it is God if I know I did not think of it. So God gave me this idea "Let's live where God wants us to live." We both agreed and this was the first major break-through in our marriage resurrection.*

Through God's help, we were able to do what we could not do on our own, and it started with making a commitment of our lives to him and then to our marriage.

VAL: *That year we committed ourselves and our marriage to the Lord. We did everything we could to build our marriage on his solid rock foundation. We became active members of a church and hosted a home group. We both participated in a Christ centered 12-Step program of recovery. We each employed our own psychologist, and worked with a Christian marriage counselor, together. We did everything we knew of to learn how to grow closer to God and closer to each other. And after one year from the time we were on Molokai, we brought the same pastor and his wife back to Molokai with us where they performed a marriage vow renewal ceremony celebrating the Lord's resurrection in our marriage!*

MARK: *We have been married for 19 years in June. We continue our commitment to Jesus. We daily pray and read the Bible together; we put time and effort into our marriage, participate in Christian recovery groups and host home Bible studies. We even put on marriage retreats, like the one advertised in today's bulletin, with no income for us, only the opportunity to invest more effort into our marriage.*

We love to tell others what God has done because He wants us to. In Mark 5:19, Jesus tells the man that he healed to, "Go home to your own people and tell them how much the Lord has done for you, and how he has had mercy on you." Telling our testimony helps us remember what is was like and what Jesus is able to do. We never want to forget how through his resurrection power he transformed our lives and our marriage. We never want to go through that difficult time in our lives again. When we remember what He has done, it feeds our faith during other struggles that we encounter in our daily lives – and we do have struggles. However, there is nothing too great for God to fix.

Whether you are struggling now or do struggle with the same or similar issues, our prayer is that this story will give you hope not in this world, but in a God who we celebrate today as having all power over all evil... RESSURECTION POWER!

Thank you and God bless!

Entry 18
Indy 500 and the "Miss America Dream"
The Indianapolis 500

Today I want to write about the Indianapolis 500 experience. I do not want this to get away from me without some recording of the appreciation and awe I feel having been part of it. Additionally, the precious lady who helps me with my house cleaning, (Opuulani Kekua), just this week noticed our newly hung pictures from our trip. She asked me if they were pictures from when we were in high school or college. (What a compliment that was!) Just for perspective, let me state that we left for Indianapolis on May 19th and returned to Kauai on May 31st of this year, 2009.

By way of introduction, let me explain that the Purdue University All American Marching Band is the "Official Band" for the Indianapolis 500. They have served in this capacity for 90 years. The year of 2009 is the centennial year of the Indianapolis 500. The administrators for the festival and race decided to honor the Purdue Band by inviting their Alumni Band to participate. I am an alumnus of Purdue University, and also of Purdue's Marching Band, having performed as their 13th "Golden Girl." In order for you to understand the enormity of the honor involved in returning to Indiana, and participating as a member of the Purdue Alumni Band at the Indy 500, I will need some leeway for digression.

As I tell this story of my baton twirling passion and heart's desire, I believe you will discover evidence that God's timing is perfect. I have told this story so many times that I have lost count. It is one that I will always treasure.

My "Miss America" Dream

I was born into a family of Purdue University people. My father, J.D. Ludwick, graduated from Purdue in 1958 with a Ph.D. in Chemistry. My mother, Jo Ludwick, spent four years working to put him through school, sometimes working two jobs. One of her jobs was Assistant to the Director of the Purdue Health Center, Mr. Fred Willis. My parents were sports fanatics, and through my mother's association with Fred, they attended every home football game. The All American Marching Band, led by the "Internationally famous Golden Girl," with her baton twirling expertise and glamorous presence, performed at every game. The Golden Girl may have been famous internationally, but she was a household name in our family. I began hearing about her before I knew what a baton was.

[For a history of the Purdue Golden Girl, see: http://www. purdue.edu/bands/goldengirl/alStory.htm]

Most little girls growing up in the United States during the 1960's aspired to be "Miss America," and they would dress up as the crowned queen of beauty. My "Miss America" dream" was to be the Golden Girl of Purdue University and lead the All American Marching Band. At 8 years old, I would organize Woodbury street parades in Richland, Washington, where I grew up. Neighbor playmates; Betty, Carol, Lisa, Jan and sister June, appeased me by grabbing pots to bang, horns to blow, and bikes to ride, while I used the baton my mother had purchased at a local department store when they had a "fire sale." (An actual fire had damaged much of the merchandise, so everything was discounted.) I frequently lead this little marching band of angels down Woodbury Street. I have often marveled at how NONE of those little gals ever once protested that I was always the leader...not once!

I actually began twirling lessons after a year of waiting to be accepted into Pat Aichele's baton twirling group. I was introduced to the idea of taking lessons by Kim, a classmate in the third grade, who performed a twirling routine for "show and tell time." My mother contacted her teacher, Pat, but was informed that classes had already begun for that season, and I would need to wait until the following year if I still desired to take lessons. I continued the Woodbury Street parades, and when the time came, I joined in Pat's classes.

I began lessons in Pat's garage when I was almost ten years old. By the following fall, my sister June decided to take lessons too. Together, we learned how to spin, twist,

toss, flip, maneuver, lunge, dance and many more movement strategies involved in the sport/art of baton twirling.
Pat placed us immediately into performing for community
parades and all kinds of events such as 7th inning stretches
of little league baseball games, talent shows, and recitals.
We learned how to present ourselves with confidence while
still having a great time. Pat held "USTA" (United States
Twirling Association) sanctioned competitions for the Tri-
City area in Washington, and it was at my first competition
that I learned how competitive I really was. I was judged on
my Solo, (one-baton twirling), and Strut routines, (marching
as if in a parade), and earned two trophies! They were both
2nd place trophies. Once I realized that somebody else had
won the 1st place trophies, I internally vowed that next time,
I would be better, and win the 1st places. Ahhh...if only it
were that simple.

In a sport where judging is involved, the subjective
perception of an individual dictates what exactly will be
expected, recognized and ultimately rewarded. The old
adage, "What doesn't kill you will make you better," applied
to us whenever we were "judged" to be less proficient than
we expected to be. It did not kill us, maybe it hurt a bit,
but it motivated us to dedicate more time and effort into
learning and perfecting our routines. By the time I was 15
years old, June and I had won many first places, lots of State
and Regional Championships, as well as several National
Championships, in 1-Baton as well as 2-Baton Twirling categories, at both major baton twirling organizations, USTA
and NBTA, (National Baton Twirling Association), competitions. In fact, we both were recognized as being most proficient at twirling multiple batons, a talent that I have always
been very grateful to God for.

During the first five years of my twirling career I went
from practicing 15 minutes per day to two hours per day
during the school year, and 6-8 hours per day throughout

the summer. It became a way of life for the Ludwick family. During my third year of competition, Pat transferred responsibility for my career to Mr. Chet Jones from Portland, Oregon. Chet taught me how to twirl…and how to win. June and I took lessons from him for about seven years, and we continued affiliation with his camps as athletes and teachers, for many more. He was a major influence on my development as a person as well as a baton champion. Chet use to tease me, using my profound but subdued sense of competitiveness, by telling me that he was going to give my "rival" the twirling tricks that I did not practice and "get down," (master the material). This, naturally, was a challenge to me. I do not believe he ever had to give any material away, once he tossed that hat into the arena.

He was probably the most creative individual I have ever met, and I will forever be grateful for his dedicated efforts to mold me into a champion. I switched teachers twice in my later career, mostly for political reasons. Even though the aspect of playing the politics never really panned out, I had the privilege of learning very different styles from Mr. Dale White from Xenia, Ohio, and Mr. Jerry Alvarez, from Fresno, California. Each of these incredible men contributed something unique to my development as a seasoned baton twirler, and prepared me for what was to come.

My 6th grade teacher, Jim Perryman, recalled that in his class, I would write about my ambition to become Purdue's Golden Girl. During every USTA Competition the official music that played over and over and over again, was actually recorded by the Purdue University All American Marching Band. In fact, Selita Sue Smith, Purdue's 8th Golden Girl, was on the cover of the USTA record album. I wanted to be like her and I was not shy in telling my friends and family that someday, I would be.

Entry 19
Friends

I will attempt to illustrate the kind of friends that I had throughout my lifetime, by sharing with you something that happened during the summer before my cancer diagnosis. My long time buddies, Debbie (Hall) Hebert, Tami (Ufkes) Schendell and Kathy (Huckleberry) Burr, invited me to take an Alaska Cruise for a foursome reunion after almost 30 years. I really do not think it is any accident that we had that chance to re-connect in May of 2007. I remember saying over and over, we are *so* blessed to be able to do this physically, financially and most importantly, we all *wanted* to reunite! These elementary school friends walked through the cancer journey with me, as well as another physical trial I had upon returning from the cruise. (I had an angioplasty performed to open up circulation in my left leg.) I believe they would have been there anyway, but it was very convenient having all their cell phone numbers programmed into my phone from the cruise!

My friends never chastised me for "always being in the gym" or "forever going to lessons and competitions" and never having much time to spend with them. They always seemed to know when I was going to be around, and planned to include me whenever they could. Believe me, it was through their efforts that our friendship was sustained. I remember one evening when Tami and Debbie pranced in our front door announcing, "Mr. and Mrs. Ludwick, we are *taking* Val!" Yes, they took me. They apparently were *fed-up* with me hiding out in my room, doing homework alone, or listening to my record player, during times that we could have been out making mischief together! Off we went, to meet Kathy and engage in potential trouble making!

During our Cruise, some of the fondest memories I have involved consensus recall of our childhood monkey business. As we remembered the individual experiences, we pointed at the gal who we believed was the instigator. As I recall, it was usually Debbie...or was it Tami...or maybe Kathy...Oh well, what I do know is that it generally *wasn't me*! (Ha-Ha ladies!! It's my journal!)

I had a few other childhood friendships, like Jeanne (La Croix) Grant, who tried out for cheerleader as my partner each of my three attempts. I was selected once in Junior High and once in High School but Jeannie never was. I am certain that she was as happy for *me* as she would have been if she had made it, Jeannie is just that type of person. I still treasure her selflessness, as I did back then. Another friend I recall being close to was Robin Boasen. Robin and I had much in common, as we were both competitive athletes. She was a gymnast, and proficient enough to win a State Title our senior year in High School. We spent a lot of time together while practicing in the Richland High gymnasium.

There were others over those early years, but I could spend eons telling stories of my lifetime of friendships and the related experiences. Suffice it to say that I have been very blessed with people who have stuck with me, encouraged me, listened and supported me in my dreams. I believe they really did dream *with* me, and when I would achieve, a part of them assimilated the victory. Maybe this is as it should be. We really do *not* become successful on our own, but achieve based upon a collage of support contributed by those who love us.

Entry 20
Family

It is HIGH TIME that I wrote about my family. Yesterday was Father's Day. I read this article in the "Daily Bread."

June 21, 2009 RBC Ministries, "Daily Bread"
<u>*Our Legacy*</u>
Children are a heritage from the Lord. —Psalm 127:3

A friend of mine wrote recently, "If we died tomorrow, the company that we are working for could easily replace us in a matter of days. But the family left behind would feel the loss for the rest of their lives. Why then do we invest so much in our work and so little in our children's lives?"

Why do we sometimes exhaust ourselves rising up early and going late to rest, "eating the bread of anxious toil" (Ps. 127:1-2 ESV), busying ourselves to make our mark on this world, and overlooking the one investment that matters beyond everything else—our children?

Solomon declared, "Children are a heritage from the Lord"—an invaluable legacy He has bequeathed us. "Like arrows in the hands of a warrior are children born in one's youth" (v.4) is his striking simile. Nothing is more worthy of our energy and time.

There is no need for "anxious toil," working night and day, the wise man Solomon proclaimed, for the Lord does take care of us (Ps. 127:2). We can make time for our children and trust that the Lord will provide for all of our physical needs. Children, whether our own or those we disciple, are our lasting legacy—an investment we'll never regret. — <u>*David H. Roper*</u>

Our children are a heritage,
A blessing from the Lord;
They bring a richness to our lives—
In each, a treasure stored. —<u>*Fasick*</u>

Time spent with your children is time wisely invested.

My father and my mother invested in me. They spent time with me, encouraged me, teaching me about the inevitable battles of life and preparing me to *win*. They taught me the truth behind what would ultimately be my favorite scripture:

Philippians 4:13, NKJV, "I can do all things through Christ who strengthens me."

Although my dad did not practice his Jewish faith, he allowed my mother to bring us up in Central United Protestant Church of Richland, WA. June and I were "trained up" in the word of God, and both of us eventually made the commitment to turn our lives over to him, accepting his reconciliatory provision of Jesus. Ultimately, we all came to know the Lord, including my father. (What an incredible Blessing to know my entire family will be there, together, in heaven someday!)

I really cannot describe the agony that I put my parents through, and really, my sister also. Not the typical strife you might anticipate in progressing through adolescence, but something I believe to be much more demanding: competitive baton twirling. Year after year they endured the disappointments and celebrated the victories, in "bi-polar" fashion. This year Mark and I gave an unusual Father's Day card to my dad. It had the hands of a professional football player, with wounds taped up, sweat dripping, and a multitude of gashes pictured. On the inside it said; "Success is knowing you did your best." We wrote on the inside an acknowledgement that dad had indeed, done his best...and has the permanent parenting scars to show for it.

My dad was the epitome of success at whatever he chose to put his efforts into. He was a brilliant nuclear chemist, an accomplished entrepreneur and a *champion maker*. His intense passion for perfection, combined with an incredibly sharp analytical mind, gave him a clear awareness of what was needed for us to be molded into winners. He spent countless hours at the gymnasium with us, coaching and prodding us into doing our routines, "just one more time." He has never been the typical father, and I have benefited tremendously because he so proficiently modeled "atypicality." The quote beside my senior high school picture illustrated my adoption of this concept. It was adapted from the poem by Robert Frost, and read: "I took the road not taken, and that has made all the difference." Here is the poem in its entirety:

The Road Not Taken

Two roads diverged in a yellow wood,
And sorry I could not travel both
And be one traveler, long I stood
And looked down one as far as I could
To where it bent in the undergrowth;
Then took the other, as just as fair
And having perhaps the better claim,
Because it was grassy and wanted wear;
Though as for that, the passing there
Had worn them really about the same,
And both that morning equally lay
In leaves no step had trodden black
Oh, I kept the first for another day!
Yet knowing how way leads on to way,
I doubted if I should ever come back.
I shall be telling this with a sigh
Somewhere ages and ages hence:
two roads diverged in a wood, and I —
I took the one less traveled by,
And that has made all the difference.
(Robert Frost)
From <u>Mountain Interval</u>, 1916, (Public Domain)

My mother was her strong, grace-filled self throughout my competitive career. She always took the "guff" I dished out as I prepared to take the stage. I never knew why I yelled and fought with my poor mother, who always ignored the onslaught in those heated moments prior to competitions. She just continued to brush my hair, pinning it securely, making sure my costumes were clean and beautiful, and all the while, she kept track of when my time to perform was. Pulling from my training in psychology, I believe that targeting my mom was a safe way to vent the anxieties I experienced.

Mom focused her competition-related inner turmoil into dedicated searches in parking lots of the competitive arenas. Her goal was always to secure a stray "lucky penny," one for me and one for June. With her determination, I believe she was never denied. Mom was a backbone for our non-traditional family. Her quiet and graceful strength provided us a place of stability to rejuvenate, and to gear up for the next challenge facing us. If there is any graciousness or generosity in my personality, it most likely came from my mother. She always was a remarkable woman, and she still is.

My parents were extraordinary in their support of my dreams. They both have influenced me tremendously throughout my life, and continue to do so. I will be forever grateful to God for placing me in their care for this lifetime.

And now let me tell you about my precious sister, June. When she decided to begin taking baton twirling lessons, I thought of it as an intrusion. Once again, my little sister was copying me, and getting support from mom and dad to do so. Oh what tremendous blessing I would have missed out on had her decision ever changed! As we went through the highs and lows of competition, we always seemed to know that there was another in the world who shared our joy, and our disappointment. Someone who really understood, because they were there when:

69

… we would throw our batons *at* one another during practices, (another way of venting that frustration and anxiety).

…we jumped on the trampoline in Jason Lee Elementary School gymnasium, and got caught by the principal, (who promptly banned us from using the gym for two weeks, and then required parental supervision).

…June finally, after several unrewarded attempts, (yet deserved, in *my* opinion!), won the "Miss Washington of Baton Twirling" crown and got the chance to compete at the Nationals for Miss America of Baton Twirling.

…we twirled under the street lights into the late hours of the evening, hoping to gain an advantage over our competitors by squeezing in just a tiny more practice time.

…we watched in horror as our faithful dad/coach attempted to demonstrate a strutting movement, laying back for the impending catch, leg out and hand outstretched, as he slipped and landed on his face, breaking a tooth.

…we sat together in the stands of Richland High School, waiting for our turn to compete at the Washington State Twirling Championships, watching midnight come and go, creating a situation that changed June from one age category to the next, (it was her birthday).

…we spent hours and hours practicing at the Ohio twirling camp, lying in the beds unable to sleep due to the incessant muscle cramps that kept us literally jumping and jerking, at times, simultaneously.

… June tossed her glasses over the edge of one arena at a National/World Competition by thrusting her hands that were clutching those glasses, forward in a futile effort to help me catch my batons. (I had just asphyxiated myself by dousing my body with acetone to help take the sweat off prior to performing. I dropped four times in the initial 30 seconds of the routine, before coming to my senses, and completed the routine without a drop...but by that time, the damage had been done!)

... the two of us would take turns standing on the sitting ledge in our front living room, holding mom's large blue vase cradled in the crook of our arm, posing for the future cameras and preparing for the day we would win a national title.

We *both* were there through it all.

There was a bond that developed through the course of these experiences that cannot be explained via words. There is a look, though. It is the look that we exchanged before I took the floor to perform what was to be, arguably, my best performance. It was at the 1979 National/World USTA Championships where I won my first of two "Champion of Champions" titles. We both knew how very hard I had practiced, and how much I wanted this one. No words were exchanged, not even a hug, just the look. It was all I needed, and I knew that I was not performing alone....I never did.

Entry 21
In pursuit of the dream

When I was a junior in high school, it was time to pursue my dream of attending Purdue University. I sent my letter of interest to the Purdue Band Department, and was shocked at the reply. Dr. Al G. Wright, famous band director of Purdue from 1954-1981 and creator of the Golden Girl position, sent me a letter of rejection. In his letter he stated that "one doesn't attend Purdue University to be the Golden Girl, she attends Purdue University to get a degree." Additionally, he emphasized that there were many champion twirlers right there in Indiana and across the Midwest, who were qualified to be Purdue's Golden Girl. After the shock wore off, I tucked something away into the recesses of my mind. It was a vision of attending graduate school at Purdue…and eventually, trying again.

I attended Central Washington University to pursue degrees in psychology and special education, bringing with me my first "Grand-National/World Championship." The USTA organization held the world's largest open baton twirling competition. They invited all countries to send representatives to compete in age categories from "0-6" through "21 and over," as well as separate one-baton, strutting, dance and twirl, two-baton and three-baton divisions, for individual athletes. Due to the unfriendly separation of the major twirling organizations, (USTA and NBTA), this competition was considered the "World Championship" by USTA members, while the NBTA members considered their national open competition to be the "World Championship." I actually determined that I would try winning both USTA and NBTA "World Championships" in the categories I was known for, multiple-baton twirling. I succeeded by winning two-baton from USTA in 1977 and NBTA in 1978, and three-baton from both organizations, (within the division of "show twirling" for NBTA), in 1978. Additionally, I won the category of USTA "Champion of Champions," (1980 and 1981), a division specifically for past Grand-National Champions, using one, two and three batons. My student, protégé and friend, Cindy Campbell and I won the USTA Duet Championship in 1981, under the direction of sister, June. (We considered it a family affair!)

I graduated in 1981 from Central Washington University with degrees in both psychology and special education, and four *wonderful* years of twirling as the solo Majorette for Central's "Wildcat Marching Band." Our claim to fame came during my junior year when our band was invited to perform for the Seattle Seahawks / Kansas City Chiefs Monday night football game in the Seattle Kingdome. My recollection of the performance includes the Chiefs running onto the field surrounding me while I was futilely trying to get to the side-lines. To this five-foot one inch female, they appeared to be a team of *giants*!

Upon graduation from Central, I once again decided that it was time to apply for acceptance at Purdue. This time I knew I needed to secure a way to fund what would be a graduate education. I was interested in counseling, so I sent in my application to the School of Educational Counseling.

A few months later, I received a rejection letter in the mail. I decided that God must be directing me to work before attending any graduate school, so I went through the process of obtaining a job using my Central Washington University degrees. I spent a year at Kennewick High School in Washington State, living at my parents' home, and teaching in a special education classroom for behavior disordered and learning disabled high school students.

What an incredible experience *that* was! I felt blessed to have been adopted into one of the best special education systems in the state, as awarded by the Washington Teaching Association. At one point early in the year it became clear that the seasoned teachers within special education did not take kindly to my "personal, relational approach." They actually held a meeting along with the school counselor, voicing their concern, and telling me that if I wanted to "do counseling" then I should go back to school and learn how. Interesting… my sentiments exactly! I proceeded to apply once again, to the Educational Counseling Program at Purdue.

This time my alumnus father made a phone call to ask why I was not accepted the previous year. The answer showed a bit of negligence on my part, but I like to think of it as God determining that it just wasn't the right time yet. (I had missed the application deadline!)

I was subsequently accepted as a Masters student into the Department of Educational Counseling at *Purdue University*!!!! By the time this news arrived, my relationships at Kennewick had developed into favorable consensus: A "Don't go!" sentiment had magically developed. My approach to student education with its more intimate qualities, had gained approval and support thanks to an endorsement from the respected and loved Vice Principal, Mr. Neil Combelic. I will always remember that year at Kennewick High as a precious experience.

It was time to consider the financial part of this venture to move half way across the country. I contacted the Purdue financial aid office, and was directed to apply for a "Residence Hall Counselorship." This position included living in a dormitory, providing guidance and supervision to undergraduate students. The number of students depended on the assignment. I received an invitation to be a counselor at Shreve Hall, where I would be in charge of 58 young women on the 5th Floor of a very large, eight-story co-educational residence hall. At the time of my tenure, "co-ed" meant that one side of the dorm were men, while the other, separated by offices, lounge areas, and a cafeteria, were women. This was my kind of place! (What did I need men hanging around for, viewing the extraordinary lengths that I engaged in to create an acceptable presentation of myself...mostly for *them*!?!)

Now we were in business! I contacted the band department to find out when try-outs were for Golden Girl, and was told it would be during the registration week. Unlikely though it was, with all the meetings and gatherings required by the Shreve Hall management, it could be accommodated into my already crammed schedule. Something else of grave importance had transpired the year before within the Purdue

Band Department, something that became of paramount importance to me. Dr. Al G. Wright retired and they hired the famous, Dr. William C. Moffit to carry on the All American Marching Band tradition. It seemed to me that God had arranged all these things for my ultimate success in claiming the coveted title of Purdue's Golden Girl.

(See these websites about Dr. Moffit: http://www.purdue. edu/bands/news/080305Moffit.html and http://marching-sport.com/m/?p=267)

After discovering the try-outs would be held on the outdoor band field, I decided to practice outside one late afternoon. Hailing from Eastern Washington, I had *no* idea what was about to happen to me. In mid-routine, I heard a thunderstorm approaching from the distance. I told myself, "Keep twirling…if it rains during try-outs, you will just have to continue, so you'd better practice in it." Ha! I had *never* seen a storm approach with such speed and ferocity! By the time I was finished with my three minute routine, I was completely soaked, unable to even *see* a baton. I laughed at my ignorance and ran for cover. Subsequently I found out that there was always an alternate site for band practices, in case of threatening Midwestern weather.

Entry 22
Learning about the AAMB

It was nice and sunny the day try-outs were held. Since I considered myself to be a competitive athlete, I wore a black and gold costume, matching Purdue's school colors. I was the only one in a "tutu!" (This is name I use for describing the glittering body suits we wore at competitions.) Everyone else got the memo that shorts were the acceptable attire. This wasn't starting out as I desired…

My performance went fine; I knew how to twirl. Many other girls took their turns, and then they announced Purdue's

12th Golden Girl…Miss Sally Betina, a senior from Marion, Ohio. She was lovely, truly a lady of grace and style.

When I first came to Purdue in 1982, I really believed that I understood what it meant to be Purdue's Golden Girl. When I tried out that year and was not chosen, Dr. Bill Moffit took me aside. He asked me to take the time, over the ensuing year, to "watch the Golden Girl, and Purdue's All American Marching Band." He recognized something that I did not. Something that I would be learning over that year, as I followed the band, examining them as they performed and represented Purdue University.

My background in competition twirling, lead me to believe that the more proficient I became in the sport, the better performer I would be, period. My image of twirling for the band involved nothing more than a highly decorated "competition twirler." The manifestation of this image was demonstrated by my appearance, including my exhibition of an extra 20 lbs. of weight. (On a five foot one inch body, this was pretty significant.) Additional indications of my ignorance seeped out in the clothes I wore, (sweat suits were my favorite attire), the way I fixed my hair, (the ever so "attractive" *bun*…to keep my hair out of the way of my baton movements), even influencing my attitude, interactions with others, and the way I carried myself.

As I studied the Golden Girl, and the All American Marching Band, what I began to realize started to reshape my original "image." I noticed many definable characteristics as well as some intangibles. Here is a non-comprehensive list off the top of my head:

• There was a *pride* that radiated from *every* member of the Purdue All American Marching Band. I saw it in the way they stood tall, marched with confidence, practiced and practiced and practiced to build an *excellence* rather than simply participating.

- It seemed that the auxiliary members were under the impression that they were achieving something higher than any competitive win! It was a culmination of all the years of practicing a "sport" (or an instrument) interwoven within the context of performance, skill exhibition and entertainment. Most definitely something *more*.
- I began to understand that there was a *responsibility* involved. This stemmed from the massive amount of people who clamored for autographs and photographs. They watched *every* move, picking up on and attempting to identify with the pride and excellence of this famous marching band.
- There were also some unsettling things for me to learn, having spent most of my twirling career as a competitive athlete. It began to dawn on me that there were expectations of attire that I had never been comfortable with... including majorette boots, crowns, capes, and "dressy" non-performance clothing. These members of the band were also *representing Purdue University*! Not just a band member...but a member of the All American Marching Band of Purdue University. (I get goose bumps just typing this!)

I tell people that the message I got from the band directors following my try-out was, "You are too fat, too short, too old and not blond enough to be our Golden Girl." (Every Golden Girl was required to conform to the image by displaying blond hair. I had inaccurately discerned that the summer sun had bleached my brownish-reddish hair enough to fit the bill.) After the initial disappointment subsided, I began to grasp clear directions to focus my continued efforts at achieving my dream. Over the year I watched, I studied... and I changed.

By the time I returned to Purdue in the fall of 1983, I had lost 20 pounds, "magically" lightened my hair, and fashioned a new attitude. I was still a residence hall counselor at Shreve Hall, and I had picked up a second emphasis in my Master's program in School Administration. I can remember the day I went into the offices of each Band Director, (four total), to ask permission to try-out once again, for the position of Golden Girl. The shock on their faces when they saw the amazing difference in my appearance was rewarding in and of itself. I saved my final meeting for Dr. William C. Moffit.

When I entered his office, Dr. Moffit focused his full attention on me and on what I had to say. This intense focus was characteristic of Bill Moffit, yet there was something different about this interaction. It was as if he was searching my soul to uncover the core of my identity and motivations. I began to discuss with him the things that I had learned from my year of studying Sally, culminating with presentation of my request to be allowed to try again.

Dr. Moffit's reply is fresh in my memory, "You know, Val, it will now come down to how you twirl in the try-outs." There was unbelievable joy that I know came through, as I nodded and smiled. He then said, "Did you hear what I said?" I replied, "Yes, I know that it will be dependent on how I twirl at try-outs, and I also know that *I can twirl*!"

Entry 23
Preparation for try-outs

There was about a week between the day that I left Dr. Moffit's office and the actual try-outs. I had responsibilities at Shreve Hall to attend to with students filling up the rooms of my fifth floor, but I found sufficient time to practice my routine. I had not shared with many people my intention to try-out for Golden Girl again. In fact, the only one from my Shreve Hall floor that I told was Karen Marner, a resident returning from the previous year. Karen was a unique individual, and we formed a friendship that would continue for many years.

During my first year at Purdue I had begun dating the residence hall counselor from the men's eighth floor, Bob Mahin. Bob was a wonderful, calming influence for me, as I had a tendency to be quite high strung, even anxious at times. He was a gentle, patient man who rarely lost his temper. He was very encouraging and supportive to me, especially in this effort to fulfill my dream. Bob was in Purdue's Jazz Band and most certainly the reason I chose an introductory song reflecting a jazz influence. My dad, as he always did over the years of performances, helped me record the jazz piece so it flowed directly into a song that had become my trademark over the years. I have always identified with the music from the Rocky movie, and have used it so often that when folks from the twirling world heard it from afar, they would say, "Val must be practicing!"

The actual selection from Rocky that I used was from Rocky I, entitled, "Going the Distance," by Bill Conti. It was the music played during the final rounds of Rocky's fight against his insurmountable opponent, Apollo Creed. As you watch the movie scene, you see Rocky being knocked down and punched over and over. Rocky's dogged persistence to achieve his goal of completing the fight without being knocked out, is portrayed in dramatic fashion.

(See the U-Tube clip: http://www.youtube.com/watch?v=25NmudB2fqg&feature=related).

I loved the intensity, the building of emotion that the Rocky music accomplished. I additionally treasured the message: No matter how many times you are knocked down as you pursue your dream, keep getting back up. And the notion that even a "dark horse" can win, if they are dedicated enough to go through the "blood, sweat and tears" that it inevitably takes for success. It was part of who I was, and who I wanted to be in my performances.

The evening prior to try-outs I was practicing at the band practice field, located directly across from Shreve Hall. As I went through my routine "just one more time" I realized that, truly, I was ready. I had done all that I possibly could to prepare for this over the course of my lifetime, and tomorrow would be my final attempt to fulfill what I had always known was my "Miss America dream." I was on track to receive my masters in counseling during that year, and I knew that if I was not chosen this time, I would move on to complete my doctorate at a different school. I sat down on the grass to pray.

I told God what he already knew; that I had longed for this ever since I could remember. I reminded him that I had worked so very hard, and wanted to succeed more than anything in my life. And then I said to him, "Lord, if you will give this to me, I will not let you down. I will always do my best and not take it for granted. But if you decide that it will be better for someone else to be chosen, it's OK…however, you will have to help me handle it."

Entry 24
And Purdue's 13th Golden Girl is…

The Scripture that best embodies the joy and perfection of that August day of Purdue's Golden Girl try-outs in 1983 may just be, *Psalm 118:24, NKJV*, "This is the day the LORD has made; we will rejoice and be glad in it."

For me, everything was absolutely perfect! At 3pm, try-out time, the sun was shining. It was not too warm or cool, just lovely. I had received the "memo" this time regarding the acceptable attire, and had chosen a nice but soft-spoken shorts outfit. When I drew my number to perform, I drew last…the very best position in any competition. (Going on last gives you an advantage of knowing what your competition has done prior to you, as well as providing opportunity for a final influential impression on the judges.)

As I type this, I can feel the very same "butterflies" in my stomach, that I felt that afternoon. This is a physiological phenomenon that I have learned to cognitively frame as "readiness." As I recall, there were about nine other young women who performed their try-out routines that day, vying for the title of Purdue's 13th Golden Girl. It was after about five of them had completed their routines when I noticed that the sidelines of the band field were beginning to fill up. In fact, I began to realize that I recognized the vast majority of those wonderful rooters...they were my 58 Shreve Hall fifth floor residents! Karen, my friend and second-year resident, organized the charge of support. The entire floor of young women had responded, lining the field with what felt like a demonstration of solidarity. I was flabbergasted!

As I sucked in air after losing my breath for what seemed like minutes, I became grateful that I noticed those familiar supporters in time to compose myself prior to my performance. Focusing was something I had learned over many years of competitive baton twirling, and I drew deeply on that skill as I prepared to twirl.

And then it was my turn. I heard the music begin as I danced, spun and twirled to the jazz tune. My heart leapt for joy as each toss was captured with certainty that only comes from being, "in the zone," or as I choose to refer to it, "twirling within God's anointing!" Then it boomed out of the cassette player with peak volume...the Rocky music. And I picked up my second baton. This is what I was born to do. I had spent more hours practicing all those intricate maneuvers using two batons than any other human probably ever has. It was my first love, my favorite. And I executed the routine with confidence that only comes through "blood, sweat and tears" of a million "getting back ups" and "one more times." And finally, I tossed up one of my two batons, did a gymnastic "walkover," flipping forward, one hand grabbing my third baton, and as I came upright again, tossed it into the air, effectively beginning my three baton portion, without stopping any batons. I maintained one, two or even three batons in the air at all times throughout the remainder of the routine. It was one of the few performances of my career that went exactly as practiced. And as the bells from the music rang out signaling the end of the fight for Rocky, where he had achieved his goal of "going the distance" with Apollo Creed, they brought my Golden Girl try-out routine to its successful completion.

It was finished. There was not a dry eye, as everyone was completely overcome with the emotion of the Rocky message, the perfect performance, and the amazing anointing that God had blessed me with. I remember my 58 ladies absolutely losing it, screaming, crying and cheering. Many of the current band members, and even the women who were competing against me, rushed out onto the field to give me hugs of approval and to share in the moment. It was my "Miss America dream," come true. For that one moment *I was* Purdue's Golden Girl. I realized that no matter what the band directors decided, at that particular moment, I had been given a gift, and I recall the relief and peace that settled into my being, knowing that I had done my very best. Nobody could ever take that moment from me, no matter who was ultimately chosen.

After a very brief consultation among the directors, Dr. William C. Moffit came to the center of the field to pronounce, "Purdue's 13th Golden Girl is Miss Valerie Ludwick!" There it was. The culmination of a heart's desire, unwavering focus, faith and determination, and… God's *perfect timing*!

It was everything I ever dreamed it would be, and more. Each year as the directors voted on whether or not I was to be retained, or "required to try-out again," I thanked God for his faithfulness and generosity to me. Each year they asked me back. For four years I held the position of Purdue's Golden Girl, throughout the time I was completing my Ph.D.

One of the most precious moments of my four year Golden Girl reign came in my second football season during a pre-game show. Dr. Al G. Wright served at each home football game as "Director Emeritus," conducting one song for the band. Because he was the creator of the Golden Girl position, his endorsement was very important to me. After he finished directing the song, he stood in front of the band as we completed the pre-game show by performing the Purdue Fight Song. That day I finished my customary three baton routine with a high toss and a gymnastic "walkover," gathering two batons in one hand and catching the third in the other hand as I did the splits. It was simply a nod and a smile from Dr. Wright that conveyed his message of approval. In my final year as Golden Girl, Dr. Al G. and his wife Gladys Wright invited me to be their feature performer for a European tour that they assembled and Gladys directed. (Among her many incredible achievements, Gladys Stone Wright was the first woman to be inducted into the National Band Association's Hall of Fame of Distinguished Band Conductors.) I was amazed at how God had brought us full circle, from initial rejection, to acceptance and eventual inclusion.

The complete description of what transpired over those four years is well beyond the scope of this journal. Maybe some other day…

Suffice it to say, it was the biggest honor and privilege of my life to represent Purdue as their 13th Golden Girl. It was my "Miss America Dream." I am humbled typing this, as I realize God's amazing grace in granting my heart's desire.

Entry 25
Indianapolis 500, 2009: Our Victory March!

And this May, 22 years later, I had the incredible honor of returning to represent Purdue once again, as their 13th Golden Girl. It was particularly amazing considering that one year prior I had been diagnosed with breast cancer. The opportunity unfolded in this way.

During the years I served as Purdue's Golden Girl, we performed many places around the Midwest, as well as in Japan and Europe. One of my favorite events where we had a standing invitation to perform was the Indianapolis 500. Every year the Purdue Marching Band acted as the official band for the Indy 500. It couldn't have been any better for a sport "hound" like me.

Each year the Indianapolis 500 Race draws over a quarter of one million fans from all over the world. It is the single largest one-day sporting event ...and Purdue's band is honored to be right in the midst of all the festivities! Every Memorial Day weekend the band leads the Indy 500 Parade on Saturday prior to the race. On race day, (Sunday), they march onto the track to perform and then to play the music for the traditional singing of "Back home in Indiana," and "God Bless America." The entire band is then provided tickets to view the race.

Each of the four times I participated at the Indy 500 I was most definitely in my element, and *loving it*! You can only imagine the overwhelming excitement I felt when I received the e-mail from the Purdue Band Alumni Office notifying me that we had been invited to return. The race committee had desired to honor the Purdue Band for their service over the past 90 years, and the centennial year of the Indy 500 Race was the perfect time to accomplish it. All alumni of the band were welcome, and that included *me*!

I couldn't wait to tell Mark the news when he arrived home from work. He was excited for me, and agreed that we would plan a vacation allowing us to be there. I did not wait long to get our plane reservations in order, and notify the Alumni Band Department that we would be joining in the fun. When final arrangements had been made and official sign up was open, we put in our request to stay with the band at the Indianapolis fairgrounds. We planned to ride the bus to and from the parade and race, and also to participate in any extra-curricular activities. At that time we requested that Mark be allowed to come alongside the band and hand out water, or carry extra batons, or whatever was needed. Mark was not a Purdue Band Alum, so we were absolutely thrilled when the directors of the Alumni Band asked him to carry a "Big-10 Flag" and march with the All American Marching Band! What an honor! Mark, having been affiliated with three of the Big-Ten Schools, was the perfect choice to carry one of the flags. He had completed his undergraduate degree at the University of Wisconsin, his Masters and Ph.D. at the University of Illinois, and a Post-Doc in the Department of Agriculture, at Purdue. We were set... almost.

There was a tiny matter of what I would wear. Mark's uniform was decided for him. He would don the traditional black pants with black shoes and purchase the official polo and T-shirt that was designed for most of the participants. But not me. I was a "Golden Girl." My requirements would be a bit more stringent.

You may have guessed that I was expected to sport a sequin body suit. Every "feature twirler" who returned was required to fit into their original costume. (Purdue has several feature twirling positions, including the "Golden Girl," the "Girl in Black" and the "Silver Twins." (http://www.purdue.edu/bands/aamb/auxiliaries.html)

Fortunately for me, the sugar-free diet that had become a way of life since my cancer diagnosis, had allowed me to keep trimmed down, at least enough to fit the bill. There were, however, some alterations that were imperative.

Yes, I kept my original Golden Girl costume. It was the one that was made for me the week that I was named to the position, and the very same one that I used for each and every performance over the course of my first two years. After all those hundreds of performances, not to mention the 22 years of resting in my Golden Girl memorabilia box, the poor old thing had atrophied substantially. When I first discovered it, I decided maybe it would be best to just have another one made. Easier said than done in the middle of the Pacific Ocean on an island where there are *no* baton twirlers.

Then one day about two months before the 500, I was walking by a local park, and noticed a little girl who was wearing a gold sequined jacket. As I connected with her and her lovely mother, it became clear to me that this was my direction from God. The woman just happened to be the director for a Kauai "Praise Hula" group, and she offered to contact her seamstress for me. Hallelujah!

Her name was Mrs. Galindo, and she would ultimately end up "putting the sparkle" back into my golden costume. She painstakingly sewed each sequin that showed signs of escaping, back into the fold, and additionally added extras where there were bare spots. It glittered once again, and I was very grateful.

I kept trying it on over the ensuing week, but I just couldn't get a peace about it. You see, the rib cage was just a bit tight, and the waist and shoulders were a bit baggy. My body had seemingly rearranged itself just enough to create these unsettling alterations. Eileen Miyasato, a dear sister in the Lord from Kauai Bible Church, had made the mistake of telling me about a month prior, that if I really needed her help, she would see what she could do. Oh boy, I decided five days before leaving, that I needed to call in a favor.

Eileen had me try on my costume, and promptly determined that "We should not trust a 22 year old zipper!" Within two hours she had ripped out that zipper, put in the extra 2 inches in the rib cage, and was ready for a fitting. She ended up spending the weekend sewing sequins onto the extra material, magically finding some way of taking in the waist and taking up the shoulders…essentially re-making the thing, all in four days! What a blessing! Now I could be comfortable performing without holding my breath and worrying that at any moment, that zipper might *pop*!!

Entry 26
19th Wedding Anniversary

It is Mark's and my 19th wedding anniversary today, (June 30, 2009) so I wanted to make a note of something God put on my heart. We celebrated this past weekend, borrowing a beautiful cabin at Kokee State Park from our friends, (Jim and Katie Cassel). Today, however, is officially our anniversary. It just reminds me of how very far that God has brought us, and how incredibly grateful that I am, just to *be*. Anniversaries have the tendency to provoke this type of reflection, but for me, cancer has intensified this process. Fortunately, it has also intensified my gratefulness to God. Amazing how God uses *all things*, even cancer, to teach us about his power, his faithfulness, and ultimately to draw us closer to him. We are planning to hold our regular weekly home group tonight. It is called, "Living Jesus Out Loud." Maybe there will be an opportunity to share this insight with whoever God chooses to bring to our little group tonight…

Entry 27
God numbers the hairs on our head

On with the Indy 500 story! Our trip was solidified and we were ready. I was just about to *pop* with excitement, and was telling everyone that I could manage to bend an ear about it. We had decided to name this our "Victory March," illustrating the incredible healings that God did to make it possible. As I have previously mentioned, if this opportunity would have transpired at any time in the past five years, I would not have been able to participate. I believe God knew my heart's desire, and he planned it, in my lifetime, at a time when I was able!

On our trip we visited our old and very dear friends, Rick and Diana Mooreland. They ran our Vineyard Church home group that we belonged to for over ten years back when we lived in Indiana. The Moorelands live just outside of Indianapolis now. What a blessing it was to see them again. And *wow*, what timing! Diana had been diagnosed with breast cancer just after I was given the thumbs up regarding my healing. It was God ordained that we would be walking through this season of our lives together.

I want to tell you about something that happened when the four of us were browsing around the Indianapolis marketplace. We had just turned the corner starting down a row of booths that were displaying their wares, when Diana and I had our attention drawn to the same item. It was a wig. You see, Diana's cancer was deemed to be much more aggressive than mine was, and she had lost her hair over the course of two rounds of chemotherapy.

The wig was a beauty, and when I asked Diana if she might like to try it on, she said that she would. I turned to the lady who was in charge of the booth, and asked her if the wig was for sale. She said, no, it was not, but asked why I was interested in it. I pointed at my dear friend's back, as she was engrossed in examining the wig. God moved in this woman's heart, and she changed her mind immediately upon viewing Diana's bald head. She rushed to bring the wig down from the manikin's head where she had posted it high above her other merchandise. In fact, this turned out to be the *only* wig in the entire marketplace. We decided it might be a gift from God, and when Diana put it on, that realization was confirmed. It fit her "*to a T!*"

God says in Scripture that he knows even the number of hairs that we have on our heads:

Luke 12:6-8, "Are not five sparrows sold for two pennies? Yet not one of them is forgotten by God. Indeed, the very hairs of your head are all numbered. Don't be afraid; you are worth more than many sparrows." (Also see: *Matthew 10:29-31*)

He planned for us to experience the blessing of the wig together. What an amazing, personal God we have!

Entry 28
Registration, sleeping arrangements and parade security

After our brief visit with Rick and Diana, armed with their generous supply of sheets, towels and blankets, Mark and I headed for check in at the Indianapolis fairgrounds. As we approached the dormitory it was all I could do to keep from screaming out loud in an effort to purge the excitement that was absolutely bubbling over inside of me. We were early and a place to sign in had yet to be established. We took our belongings up to the rooms, checking out this "co-ed" sleeping arrangement. The President of the Alumni Band, Hank Evans, invited us to join him and six other men, in a private area that had its own bathroom. Hummmm, Mark, me, and six other men...without hesitating Mark answered,

"No, thank you!" OK, so we looked over the remaining rooms. We decided to take Hank up on his second offer, and that was to take over the only other private room, and "be picky" about who we invited to join us. We set up our bunk beds and headed down to register.

One of the first connections that I wanted to make was with June Lauer, Purdue's fourth Golden Girl, who wears many honored hats for the Purdue Band including the designation, Director of the Alumni Auxiliaries. June had been in contact with me since the announcement of the Indy 500 opportunity. She was aware of my recent cancer diagnosis. June encouraged me and assured me that whatever I would be able to accomplish during our performances would be sufficient. As the time neared for our trip, June e-mailed me to inform me that there would be plenty of water alongside the route, in case I needed it.

When I had difficulty procuring a gold sequin costume, June immediately sent out an "APB," requesting help from the Purdue band family. She told me that if we did not find something suitable, then she would take my measurements to a seamstress and have a new costume made back in the Midwest! I recognized that I was only one of the many auxiliary members she was dealing with, as she was in charge of everyone from flag carriers and dancers to banner carriers and other baton twirlers. She did an amazing job of handling the various issues that cropped up, including remembering to secure a "body guard" for security purposes.

When I was a member of the band back in the "dark ages"....we always had people who marched alongside us, dutifully watching for signs of potential trouble. There was only one time when it was necessary for my designated protector to assist me. It was at an away football game with our arch rivals, Indiana University. I was grateful for the swiftness of the body guard intervening when an obviously drunk Indiana fan rushed toward me, shoving me in a purposeful attempt to knock me down. He was tackled and promptly escorted to the police by our Purdue band security with the help of a couple of our faithful drum line dudes.

Now that I am on the subject, there was that one other time when I was grabbed from behind while walking on the field at an Ohio State football game in Columbus, Ohio. During my very first meeting with the band staff as Purdue's 13th Golden Girl, Dr. Moffit and Glenda Freeze, (our lovely and talented Auxiliary Director), emphasized that I was expected to use my baton as a weapon, if necessary. They spelled out the danger associated with *not* reacting if I was threatened, leaving open the potential for a copy-cat fan to attack any of our band members, particularly females donning attractive costuming.

I didn't even think about it as I felt very large hands grasping me from behind. I swung my baton like a club, with as much force as I was able. As I turned to see the impact of my mighty thrust, I saw my baton crash down on the top of the head of the Ohio State mascot, "Brutus Buckeye!" I yelled, "Don't you ever do that again you big fat eyeball!" Brutus playfully acted out being hurt from my blow. In all actuality, my whack fell upon at least six inches of pillow that was part of the enormous head of his costume, providing cushioning to that point that I doubt he ever even felt it! Such were the reasons that June Lauer made certain that she obtained security for the Indy 500, and I was thankful for her diligence.

Entry 29
The Golden Girls of Purdue University

As the members of the Alumni Band came pouring in over the next couple hours, we did our official check-in and picked up Mark's uniform tops, our Purdue stickers and our souvenir pins. We connected with as many of the Alums that we could. It was during this time that I presented each of the five other returning Golden Girls with something that I had prepared especially for them.

When I found out the names of the Golden Girls who would be coming to the Indy 500, I considered what I wanted to tell each of them. I realized as I pondered that question, that I had actually *seen* each one of these special women as the Golden Girl. I could speak from experience about the unique qualities that each individual woman brought to the coveted position. After visualizing myself taking each one aside, I realized that in the midst of all the excitement, my sentiments would likely be lost and forgotten. I decided to write a letter, and give it to them when they arrived. Here is the letter I gave to each Golden Girl that day:

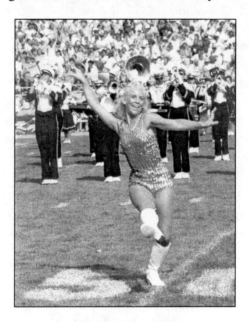

"Golden Girl Val"

Dear Golden Girls; June, Susan, Dawn, Holly, Alisha,

I wanted to tell you all that I consider it a tremendous privilege to have this opportunity to perform in this Indianapolis 500 Centennial Celebration, alongside each of you. You are all ladies of elegance and integrity, and I feel Blessed to be part of your lives this weekend.

I remember each of you with your unique qualities. Susan, a woman of sophistication, grace and style; Dawn, with your joy and spirit; Holly, emanating your genuineness and talent; Alisha, delightful and lovely and June; with your remarkable presence that commands enthusiasm and excitement. You are truly ladies worthy of admiration.

It is with inexpressible pleasure that I join you in contributing to this "Once in a lifetime" event.

Many Blessings,
Valerie (Ludwick) Willman

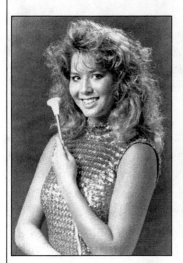

"*Golden Girl Dawn*"

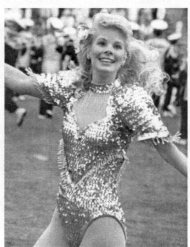

"*Golden Girl Alisha*"

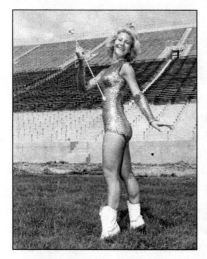

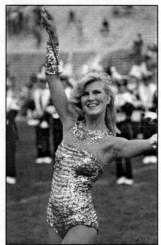

"Golden Girl June"   *"Golden Girl Susan"*

The letter brought tears from each one of the five precious ladies who would join me in representing Purdue as their Golden Girl, at the Indianapolis 500, one more time. I believe the urging I experienced to compose this letter was from

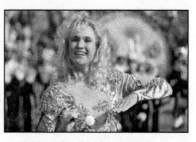

"Golden Girl Holly"

the Holy Spirit. There were perfect, God ordained reasons to write it. I believe the letter released us all to perform within our unique giftings. It allowed us freedom from competitiveness that might have otherwise spoiled our time together. And, personally, it made me feel that I was not alone. We were all together in this united objective; to perform proficiently with the grace and style characteristic of a Purdue Golden Girl. I was so very grateful to the Lord for placing the desire into my heart.

Golden Girl Biographies can be found on the Purdue Webpage at:

https://www.purdue.edu/bands/goldengirl/Welcome.html#Bios

Entry 30
Practice

Our fearless leader, Dr. William, (Bill), Kissinger, arrived and we all scuttled about getting ready for our official practice in the parking lot of the fairgrounds. Bill gave us our instructions, and off we went, around and around and around in a huge circular formation. Mark had been given the Wisconsin flag to carry, his undergraduate alma-mater, and I was paired beside Golden Girl Dawn to twirl as we proceeded down the parade route. Golden Girl Susie held the title two years prior to me, so she was considered the "Senior Golden Girl." She would lead our Alumni Band, twirling just behind our official banner. Golden Girl June had decided that she would participate by carrying the banner along with alumni Girl in Black, Lisa (Ross) Todd. I decided it was fitting that, at 50 years old, I was actually the oldest twirling Golden Girl. I was the only one who ever held the title while in graduate school.

At practice there was a certain drum cadence that was played, and all the feature twirlers had a conference regarding what we should be doing during it. Golden Girl Holly urged me to demonstrate the marching style that she remembered me for. After thinking about it, I recalled that I used to do a "high step march" very rapidly, to the unusually fast drum cadence. Naturally, I had to go ahead and try it...and boy did I regret it! At first, it was just cool, as Holly and the rest of the twirlers clapped with joy encouraging me. But, afterwards, I recognized a twang in my left thigh that didn't exist prior to my "showing off." I would deal with the anxieties that a pulled muscle elicits, into the late hours of that night.

Mark embodied the amazing trouper that I have always admired in him. He had never marched with a band in his entire life. Thrown into the middle of sarcastic comments and haughty sentiments, understandably stemming from a focus on excellence and pride that was traditionally represented within returning members of the All American Marching Band, Mark stood his ground. In fact, he marched his ground, learning to stay in step, holding the Big-10 Flag, singing "Hail Purdue" and "Honor of Ol' Purdue" while moving his right hand in time with the beat, (customarily hitting the left chest, returning to the side, and then bending the arm at the elbow, and back down to the side.) This sequence was performed every four steps.

Mark would eventually earn the respect and admiration of the entire Big-10 Flag group, and actually be asked back, "anytime the Alumni Band performs." What a man! My hero!! (Knowing for certain that this whole Indy 500 deal was *not* Mark's "cup of tea," made his willingness to come alongside me in my dream "Victory March," all the more precious.)

After practice, Mark and I cleaned up and joined the others for the dinner banquet. There were many shouts of "Hail Purdue," movies of years past, old band shows, and speeches from Hank, Bill and a few others. It was directly after dinner when I had the opportunity to meet the current Director of the Purdue All American Marching Band, Mr. Jay Gephart. I had never before met Jay, having only communicated via e-mail a couple of times. However, there was a connection that ran much deeper then would be explainable on the surface. You see, Jay's wife battles cancer. Of all the devious plans that Satan had for cancer, I do not believe he ever foretold the intimacy that is inherent within relationships of those affected by cancer. It is most certainly the manifestation of *Romans 8:28*. ("And we know that in all things God works for the good of those who love him, who have been called according to his purpose.")

Entry 31
A digression regarding Jay Gephart
Written 8/17/2009

Today I received an e-mail that deeply saddened me, yet prompted my Spirit to rejoice greatly. It was an announcement from Jay Gephart:

Carolyn Gephart loses battle with breast cancer

Dear Purdue family,
It is with deep sadness that I write this email to inform you that my beautiful wife Carolyn passed away this morning at 7:20am after a 3 year struggle with breast cancer. She was surrounded by her children and many family members when she went to be with our Lord and Savior Jesus Christ in Heaven. She took a major turn Saturday night and we took her to the hospital early Sunday morning. It was at that time we were told that she was in the final stages of her fight against breast cancer and we had days and perhaps only hours.

Carolyn fought this illness to the very end. She had a chemo treatment last Thursday and was told things were not looking good. She looked up at me and said "I am not done fighting." Little did we know what was around the corner. Nonetheless, I told you that Carolyn was my hero and I feel even more strongly about that today. She was as courageous and selfless as anyone I have ever known. God will certainly greet her with "Well done, good and faithful servant."

For those who had the privilege of knowing Carolyn, you knew where she stood regarding her faith. It was our faith and trust in Jesus Christ that sustained our family throughout this entire ordeal. Now we rejoice knowing she is in heaven and is seeing our Lord and Savior face to face. We rejoice that she has no more pain or breathing problems, no more fear or anxiety. She is seeing the glory of the Lord - faith for Carolyn is now reality.

Carolyn Frantz Gephart was the love of my life. I have tried to be strong for Carolyn and our children from the time her cancer was diagnosed. Our Purdue students, faculty and staff have played a major role in my ability to cope with Carolyn's illness. I could never have done it without them and for that I am eternally grateful. Carolyn gave me four beautiful children who loved their mother deeply. We honor her as we move forward, with Carolyn continuing to lead the charge from her place in heaven. She will be our biggest champion. I have never known anyone with a more beautiful heart than Carolyn. God gave me a gift when He gave her to me these past 26 years. We celebrated our anniversary just last Thursday. Furthermore, we know we will see Carolyn again and will live with her for eternity in heaven. As hard as this seems now, this life will seem like a blip on the eternal radar screen!

At this time, we ask that you please pray for our children. They are suffering so I ask that you pray for our family as we face the coming days and weeks. Also pray for Bouldin, Flo, Tommy and Paola - as difficult as this is for us, it is extremely hard for Carolyn's mom, dad, brother and sister-in-law.

We will post information on the Purdue band website www.purdue.edu/bands about a memorial service honoring Carolyn's life. In the meantime, please know how much I love my Purdue family. Pat Newton and Kathy Matter from the Purdue band staff will serve as my mouthpiece during the next few days.

Sincerely, Jay
(Reprinted with permission)

I immediately sent Jay an e-mail letting him know that I shared his grief. Then I reflected on what a tremendous witness that he embodied during his time of incredible loss. On an occasion when most people would probably be extremely self-consumed, Jay demonstrated his faith in Jesus by sharing with everyone on the Band Department's e-mail list. He planted seeds of hope for those who might be experiencing similar losses. What a powerful illustration of how the love of the Lord can be strength in time of weakness.

Prevailing sentiments laden with "political correctness" might inhibit such a proclamation from someone with tenuous faith, but Jay's e-mail shines forth truth without apology. I was awed and inspired by Jay's courage to seize this opportunity to live Jesus out loud. Mark and I are praying that the seeds he is planting will be cultivated, drawing innumerable precious souls to the Lord.

Entry 32
Indy 500: After the dinner reception

After the dinner banquet, Mark and I decided to make an initial attempt at turning in for the night. Outside our building were the sounds of a Drum Corp, practicing into the night, and inside the dormitory were Purdue band members milling around, laughing and sharing their excitement about tomorrow's parade. Our private room helped. Although we did not end up rooming with all men, we did end up with all women... and Mark! (There also was rumor of a man who came in after we were all asleep, and left before we awoke, utilizing the one open bunk bed.)

I wanted to include a funny side note here. It involved one of the female band members who joined us in our private room. When she put her stuff onto a bunk, effectively laying a claim on it, she noticed my three batons leaning onto the edge of my bed. She found it necessary to say to me, that when she saw those batons, she knew her chances of getting into the bathroom in the morning were slim to none. (We twirlers evidently carry the reputation of hogging available mirror space, excessively primping and curling! You would have to ask my roommates if I upheld this time honored tradition.)

As I slid under my borrowed sheet and blanket, I recognized the incessant burning emanating from my thigh. After attempting to sleep for about an hour, praying fervently for healing, I finally surrendered to God's prompting for me to get some ice to place on that darned pulled muscle. The burning stopped long enough for me to get to sleep, and in the morning, it was no longer an issue. Just one more miracle I received through answered prayer, and obedience.

Entry 33
The Victory March

Ahhhhh, *the* morning finally arrived! It was the Saturday of the Indianapolis 500 Parade, and we were going to be *in it*!!! Unreal! I left my room still clothed in pajamas to get a drink of water, and was met by a video camera in my face. I could not believe it! Who dare film me before I had even wiped the sleep from my eyes? They were asking me questions too. I had forgotten this aspect of band life, or should I say, life as the Golden Girl? Everywhere we went there were band members wanting pictures with the Golden Girls and that did not cease as we arrived via busses at the parade waiting area. I wondered for a brief moment whether I was getting too old for this sort of attention, but the thought quickly passed, dissolving into a familiarity stemming from the four years of celebrity, albeit 22 years ago.

There was still a tiny matter that I needed to attend to before we took off down the parade route. I needed someone to carry my extra batons! Because I was known for my multiple baton twirling expertise, I wanted to demonstrate it as much as I could, during the parade. I feared that I would not be able to march the entire two miles while twirling two or three batons, so I looked for a willing carrier. It was our security guard, Bob Pullan who graciously agreed to serve my need. He had secured a "manly" carrier, borrowing a black violin case to place extra batons in. (He said it was not masculine to be carrying just batons, but the violin case transformed the appearance, creating a "macho" exterior!)

I recognized that the Indy 500 Parade traditionally began by traveling past a grandstand area. In that area were all the television cameras. The road is lined with black and white checkered carpeting, making perception, including ability to see batons spinning, a bit tricky. After much internal debate, I decided to go for it and begin the parade with my favorite, two batons.

As we began marching, the tears welled up in my eyes. It was really happening. I was marching in the Indy 500 Parade. It was my "Victory March," and I praised God from the time I began until the final steps. As we marched by the grandstand, I realized that God had allowed me to be on the side of the announcers…and the T.V. cameras. I saw one camera focused directly on me, and I went into action, playing to the crowd and that camera. All the way through the notoriously difficult parade, I twirled, I sang, I pointed to the sky giving deference and praises to God. It was most definitely a dream come true.

(See: http://www.youtube.com/watch?v=rdcaRF7_fPw at minute 5:40).

About half way through the parade route, we were offered bottled water. I had mentioned to my sister, June, that this was something I would probably need to succumb to, being the "older athlete!" She just said, "Well, Val, why don't you just twirl with one hand and drink with the other?" I remembered her saying this as I went for my drink. I never stopped my left hand, moving the baton through my fingers over and over again, just like we used to do at competitions while chatting with one another. The crowd seemed to appreciate it, and I enjoyed the challenge of drinking while twirling!

It was at the point in the parade that only two more blocks remained, when I finally gave up my second baton. Bob dutifully grabbed it and secured it in the violin case. Had I known that there were only a couple blocks left, I would not have found it necessary to surrender one of the batons, but I had no way of knowing how much further the end was, and man, was I getting tired!

It was only at the end of the parade when I realized that God had given me a gift that I had not even thought possible, so I never asked for it. I did not drop. The entire two miles of parade, I never had to pick up a baton. What a blessing! The focus the Lord gave me was something I had prayed for, and he must have just wanted to give me an extra special present. I was so very grateful. I didn't have to wonder if anyone snapped a picture at just the wrong moment, as I was running for a misbehaving baton on the loose, or if I would see my "hiney" on the front page of a newspaper with the caption, "nobody's perfect,"…there just weren't any drops!

Everyone seemed ecstatic afterwards. A few people left our group to connect with their families, but most rode the bus back to the fairgrounds.

When we were finished changing from the parade, we were notified that a laptop with pictures from the parade was playing a slideshow in the lounge area. We hustled down the hall to take a look. Our Purdue alumni photographers had done an awesome job capturing the experience in two dimensions.

As I was enjoying the show, a picture of the undergrad AAMB appeared on the screen, obviously taken from the top of a building. A strong emotion of pride swept over me as I noticed the straight lines of marchers, all stepping with the same foot in synchrony. I thought to myself, now that's my All American Marching Band! And then it dawned on me...if this picture of the undergrad band had been taken, surely there would be a similar picture of *us*!! I remember the dread spreading across my brain, as I prayed, "Please God, let us look at least similar to them. We tried so hard. Oh please God!" And then, the photo appeared, and I gasped in glee! We had just as straight lines, we were all in step, and if you traded our uniforms for theirs, you would not have been able to detect a difference! How incredible was *that*?! I believe that picture illustrated the pride and excellence that is embedded within the fabric of Purdue's All American Marching Band. It never leaves you.

Entry 34
Race Day

The race day wake-up call for our room was 4:30a.m. At about 3a.m., I had to go to the bathroom. I tried to be very quiet, but apparently, not quiet enough. I woke up one of the ladies in a top bunk, who promptly jerked herself straight up in bed, screaming, "What time is it? Is it time to go?" Inside I was laughing hysterically, as I recognized her anxiety about missing the bus that was scheduled to leave the fairgrounds at 5a.m. We all were very aware that if we missed the bus, we would not be going to the Indy 500.

This has always been the policy of the band, and we had been drilled over our years at Purdue with this threat of impending doom related to potentially blowing it by arriving late, reaping our consequence of abandonment. (Only once did I cut it close, only to find myself running for Bus #1, completely at the mercy of our Director, Bill Moffit. Yes... he stopped, and I got to go on the trip! *Whew*!) I quietly assured this unsettled woman that it was not yet time to wake up, and that she could try to get a little more sleep.

I cannot speak for anyone else, but when my alarm went off, strategically set about 10 minutes prior to everyone else, I shot out of bed with the speed and alertness that might be expected from downing a couple shots of espresso. It was *race day*!!!

Once we were all loaded onto the busses, it was the old game we were all too familiar with, "hurry up and wait." The reasoning behind getting us old-folks up and running, eight hours before the race, was to beat the traffic. This is always a huge factor to be considered when dealing with Indy 500 traffic, involving over half a million people. The Purdue band busses never tried doing this on their own. They always arranged a police escort for the morning of the race. The catch was that the escort rendezvoused with all the bands performing at the track at about 6a.m. This allowed the entire group of busses to arrive at the track in plenty of time to get ready to… well, to wait! And we waited. And we waited. There were rumors that we would be going onto the track at about 10a.m., but it turned out to be about 9:30a.m. Good thing we were ready!

As we went through the tunnel taking us through the back side of the stands on the fourth turn of the race course, I once again felt my throat choking up, and my eyes watering. "Here we are. It really is happening," I told myself. "Thank you Lord!"

And then we stepped onto the track…and we lost our breath. It's not what you think. We actually couldn't believe our eyes. *Nobody was there*! I am not joking here. Apparently what had changed since we all had marched in the 500, was the start time. But, what had not been altered was *our* start time! I remember the other twirlers looking around and at each other, and finally I shouted, "Let's do it for the Lord!" There were several confirming voices, and off we went, down the Indy 500 track, twirling and singing and yelling to the very few fans that were already in their seats, thanking them for coming early to see us.

Aside from that little disappointment, it was pretty surreal. After all, we were on the same track where, within a few short hours, the famous Indianapolis 500 Race would be taking place! We marched around turn four, and down the straightaway just past the "start-finish line." At that location there were a few more people who had congregated to see the band. And then, it was over. We were ushered into the infield, and we walked back to our busses with the memories of this "once in a lifetime" experience.

Our "Victory March" was complete. For me, it was substantiation of God's miracle of healing in my life. Mark and I praised God for his unbelievable grace in allowing us to participate. We had made new friends and connected with old buddies. It was a remarkable experience and we were so very grateful to those individuals who made it possible, especially President of the Purdue Alumni Band Organization, Hank Evans, and Director of the Alumni Auxiliaries, June Lauer.

Entry 35
First e-mail to Victory over cancer list

I am reading the Daily Bread's version of the One Year Bible. There are commentaries associated with the New Testament readings. Today's commentary of the reading from *Acts 16* had the following insight:

"... often our personal world has to be shaken up by the onset of a life-threatening disease, a divorce, a vocational or financial reversal, before we consider the really important questions in life."

It prompted me to review the questions that I was confronted with while plodding along my cancer journey. This channeled my realization that God is guiding me to tackle the sequence of e-mails that Mark and I sent to our, "Victory over cancer" list. These e-mails provide a fairly clear outline of our journey through cancer. Very interesting how God used this commentary as a vehicle for prompting!

Here we go...

E-mail #1

Date: Mon 05/12/08 05:34 PM

Dear friends and family:

We are sending out this e-mail to share with you that God is bringing us into a new arena of challenge. On Monday (5/5/08), Val was diagnosed with "infiltrating ductal carcinoma." We are told that this is the most common and treatable form of breast cancer. This week has been filled with incredible blessings, alongside the overwhelming emotions and demands that accompany this type of medical condition. Val says she learned more about breast cancer in the 24 hours post diagnosis, than she ever really wanted to know. We have been inundated with stories of hope, of victory, of God's immeasurable love and sustenance, along with opinions on treatments, books, fruits, medicines, prayers, INCREDIBLE hearts reaching out to us, as we begin this journey.

At this point, we are asking for prayer that we will stand upright with God's integrity, and hear clearly from the Lord for treatment direction. Surgery is set up for May 21, in Waimea at Kauai Veterans Memorial Hospital (KVMH) and will be performed by Dr. Emilia Dauway-Williams. Dr. Williams is a specialist in breast cancer. She has training in medical school at Johns Hopkins University and practiced in Seattle. She was voted one of the best Seattle physicians in the category of oncology. Additionally, she has personal, family experience with the disease. (It never ceases to amaze us how competent the professionals are here in this tiny little island in the middle of the Pacific ocean!)

When we spoke with Dr. Williams regarding our treatment options, we were concerned about a few engagements that we have coming up shortly and the possibility that we would have to cancel them. The first...let's get our priorities straight now, is coming up next week. The "World Championship Samoan Fire Knife Competition" in Oahu!!! We had planned to attend this 4-day event. Val asked the Doctor how soon we needed to schedule the surgery. She said that she did not want us to wait for 2 months, but 2 weeks would be fine. We looked on the calendar and came up with a wonderful fit! God gives us the desires of our heart...and that was one of ours! Then, we told her about our upcoming marriage retreat that had just been announced and advertised for June 20-21 at the Kauai Marriott Resort. She actually said, "I WANT you to do that!" We asked her if she also wanted to know more about it...and she said yes. We pulled out a brochure describing it and began to tell her about our own "Miracle Marriage" and how the Lord brought us both to our knees and restored our relationship with Him and with each other. She said, "I wanna come!" We were thrilled and believe this is one fantastic thing that God is doing through allowing this challenge.

For those of you who prefer less details, stop reading here. We love you and appreciate your prayers. Please let us know if you want to be updated through this incredible adventure the Lord is allowing into our lives! God has made us all dif-

ferent and we are aware there are some who will desire more details, so here is what we know so far:

We will need to make a decision regarding the nature of the surgery. Some of the information indicates that the lump that was discovered has been encased by Val's body and can possibly be removed via a "lumpectomy." The recommended accompanying treatment, assuming that analysis of adjacent lymph nodes shows no signs of the cancer spreading, is "radiation therapy." The most common radiation therapy is a 6 week process of exposure for 10 min. per day/5 days per week. Unfortunately, this is not available on our Island. It is available on the Island of Oahu. That is a plane ride away. The other option we are considering is for a "mastectomy." This would remove the breast, and assuming no spreading of the cancer, afford opportunity for eventual reconstructive surgery. The success rates for both of these treatment options (lumpectomy plus radiation and mastectomy) are approximately the same, with a success rate of about 98-99%. We are also considering having the lumpectomy without radiation treatment. The success rates for this process are not as well defined, but look about 75+%.

The thing about percentages and statistics is that they generally do not factor in important elements such as: personal attitude, Faith, Prayer, personality, and other social/lifestyle and Spiritual components to the healing process. We trust in Jesus Christ and His promises over any earthly "wisdom." Just a couple of the scriptures that we have been claiming:

Isaiah 54:17, NKJV, *"No weapon formed against you shall prosper, and every tongue which rises against you in judgment you shall condemn. This is the heritage of the servants of the LORD, and their righteousness is from me, says the LORD."*

Romans 8:28, "And we know that in all things God works for the good of those who love him, who have been called according to his purpose."

We love all of you, and thank you for lifting us up in Prayer. We are also praying for YOU! Remember, God NEVER allows anything into our lives without also having a purpose for it. He WILL use this for His Glory and our good.

Please let us know if you desire to receive updates and we will keep you posted as best we are able.

Aloha Blessings,

* Val and Mark *

Whew! Reading that again stirs up many emotions for me. There is the memory, and accompanying emotional pain from the initial shock of being diagnosed with cancer. There is nothing in this world that could prepare me for that moment. It was the quintessential method God used to "rock my world."

There are other emotions rumbling around inside me right now. One of them is the memory of how *overwhelming* the experience was. I remember groping for direction, pouring myself into an academic exercise of gathering as much information as quickly as I was capable of navigating the Internet. Looking back at it, I believe this gave me a direction, a sense of competence and hope, all the while pacifying my emotional overload. The bottom line for me was something I kept asking God, "What can I *do*?"

As the e-mail indicates, within 24 hours, I had collected an abundance of information on breast cancer. In that process I had learned many things including the fact that *sugar* feeds cancer cells! I believe that the message God was communicating to me was not a new one. He had been trying to let me know for years that being a "sugarholic," a term I often would use to refer to myself, was not only a *sin* for me, it was also killing me. Isn't it incredible that something as innocuous looking as sugar, used in excess, could actually kill? I believe this illustrates a point that God makes clear in his word. Anything or anyone that we "worship" or make into an "idol" becomes a sin, and leads to death. For me, clearly, it was sugar. So I stopped eating it.

There is also something very wonderful that begins to surface in my emotional memory bank as I re-experience this time in our journey. It is a confidence that no matter what we were going through, God was still in control. He had not forgotten or abandoned us. It was on a platform of faith that we established our home base for this cancer journey. It is from a position of standing firmly on this platform that we composed this e-mail…and every e-mail that followed.

Entry 36
Initial reactions

Everyone and their dog, has ideas on how to treat cancer. I believe I heard very close to all of the options for treat-ments, from eating goji berries, drinking noni juice, downing organic grasses, vitamins and supplements, performing exercise, shooting up chemicals of natural and man-made origins, fervent prayer and fasting, to doing nothing at all. I am not kidding. I could fill a page or even more with all the good-intentioned remedies with substantiation from one personal report of success to mounds of carefully controlled research projects with supporting evidence.

Believe it or not, this portion of our journey was the most exhaustingly difficult. With our already maxed out emo-tional resources, Mark and I were fielding an indefinable amount of well-meaning but intrusively passionate people offering their two cents worth, purposing to offer direction for our treatment choice. And, everyone believed that their treatment was the one where my cure would manifest. Oh my. When we filtered through the defensiveness and got out from under the overpowering wave of impending sentiments that "this is the *only* way to go," what astounding compassion and love we felt from all those incredible people. This was one of the most surprising treasures that I discovered via my cancer journey.

Another form of love and support came from personal reactions upon hearing my news. I would estimate that about 50% of those I revealed my condition to, began to cry. There was essentially no gender difference. The word cancer holds such enormous power and triggers such fear inducing associations that one would have to be from another planet to not have an intense reaction to it. Let me tell you about a few of the reactions I hold most dearly in my heart.

Reactions to my diagnosis

I will begin with Rick Mooreland. Rick is a precious brother in the Lord. He and his wife, Diana, lead the Valparaiso, Indiana Vineyard Church home group that Mark and I were members of for ten years. It was during this time that Mark and I separated. Rick acted as a protector through those two years, keeping me connected with the Lord and his plan for my life. When Mark and I left Indiana for Washington State, we were preceded by Rick and Diana, who had just relocated to Mount Vernon, Washington. Although Mark and I moved to the opposite side of the Cascade Mountains in South-Eastern Washington, the Moorelands found time to visit us regularly. Over the years, we have remained in touch so they received our initial e-mail.

When Rick called me, he sounded quite angry. He shouted through his tears into the phone, "This is *not OK* with me!"

He proceeded to illustrate his frustration by telling me about the conversations he was having with God, questioning this turn of events in my life. To me, this was a valuable reminder of how deeply our walk affects those that God has joined us with in this life. The fact that Rick lived thousands of miles away from me had little influence on his emotional connection to me and my pain. It was so funny that toward the end of our conversation, Rick stated, "I think you are doing much better with this than I am. I had better regroup here!" The fact that Rick had such a strong emotional response to *me* being diagnosed with cancer, forcing him to come to terms with God's sovereignty, was most likely part of God's plan. I believe it helped him prepare for what would soon develop in his own life. You see, directly after I was cleared of cancer and told I did not need chemotherapy, Diana was diagnosed with an extremely aggressive form of breast cancer.

One of the first calls I made was to my sister, June. She and I had been through so much as twirling buddies and remained very close throughout the years and over the miles of separation geographically. When I told her, she was very quiet. She took a matter of fact approach, most assuredly an emotional defense utilized to provide me with some semblance of support. Although you might expect this to take us into an intellectual zone that would ultimately prevent us from connecting emotionally, the opposite effect transpired. After discussing the physical ramifications of such a diagnosis, and the immediate plan to address this problem, we both felt a release from the initial hopelessness. This allowed us to turn to our common faith in Jesus, looking to him for comfort, peace and wisdom. We prayed. It enveloped us at a depth that was reminiscent of "the look" she gave me at the Grand National Baton Championships. It was the look that meant, "I know you and I am with you...in a way that nobody else could be." I was not alone.

Entry 37
Family and other reactions

My mom and dad have always been major players in my life. They were cheerleaders and coaches for me as I pursued my goals and accomplishments. Eventually, they found ways to support us even when Mark and I announced that we believed God was moving us to Kauai. (This move took us far away from their Oregon residence as well as the dream for one of their daughters to assume the Richland home that dad built and we grew up in.) It was very tough to tell them that I had been diagnosed with cancer, particularly in light of the fact that geographically, they were so far away.

I dreaded telling them the bad news, but knew I needed their loving support. I had to repeat myself several times over the phone for them to bring down their defenses enough to actually understand me. I said, "My doctor told me that I have the most treatable form of cancer," and I explained what I knew just minutes after I had been informed myself. It was hard, really hard. It wasn't supposed to be this way. I knew from my training as a psychologist that some of the most difficult stressors in life arise as parents experience their children's trials. (The ultimate example of this is death of a child.) Because cancer inevitably elicits associations with death, particularly for people in my parents' generation, this was a horrifying shock.

As in every situation that we had faced as a family, we worked through it. We focused on what we *could* do as opposed to the unknowns. We developed a plan that included my scheduled visit to my doctor for further explanation, much prayer solicitation from all of our prayer groups, and investigation of this malicious intruder, breast cancer. By the time we finished the call, I had a direction, and as I expected, I felt their unconditional support and love. Within a week my father sent me two products that he had identified via his research as helpful for treating my form of cancer; DIM (Diindolylmethane, to treat estrogen related problems) and Modified Citrus Pectin (to address metastatic potential). I cannot describe the strength and hope this elicited from within me. We were actually *doing* something to affect the development and spread of the cancer.

After my parents and sister, I called my dear friend, our Pastor's wife, Darlene Walker. I will name her reaction as one of "tears without fears." I knew she felt deeply for me and it was from this relational attachment that the tears flowed, but her fiercely determined faith overshadowed every potential fear. She shouted, "I claim this scripture for you, *Isaiah 54:17, NKJV,* "No weapon formed against you shall prosper, and every tongue which rises against you in judgment you shall condemn. This is the heritage of the servants of the LORD, and their righteousness is from me says the LORD." It has been my mantra ever since that day.

When I had my leg angioplasty in August, of 2006, my husband and I stayed in touch with my talented and personable surgeon, Dr. James Wong. He was on my initial e-mail list, and the reason I am mentioning him in this context is to describe his unpredicted response, coming moments after I had sent out the e-mail. I sent him a preliminary e-mail, letting him know that he would be receiving a mass e-mail explaining more details, but I wanted to ask his professional opinion regarding references for medical help on the Island of Oahu, where he worked. I sent him the personal e-mail and then I hit the button sending the mass e-mail. Immediately my cell phone rang. I am not kidding. I answered it, and on the other end of the line I heard, "This is James Wong....oh Val." And we sat paused for several seconds. Again, a connection I cannot explain except to tell you that it was such a comfort. How can that be? "Oh Val," was all that was said. It was all that was needed. Of course he had several recommendations and encouragements to share with me after the initial connection, but it is in the moments of silence where sharing of pain occurred, where expression of the inexpressible actually transpired. It is a moment that I will always remember, and treasure.

I have a friend from my years in Indiana that I have counted as a sister. Nikki Fitzgerald has walked beside me through the tough times of Mark and I being separated and has shared her own life struggles through the years. I received one of the greatest tributes ever from Nikki and her husband Jerry, for my 50th birthday this past October. They determined that they would declare and institute something they named the "50 Days of Val!" On my birthday and for the succeeding 50 days, they took turns contacting me. They used e-mail, sent care packages, and made phone calls for 50 days in a row! (Talk about dedication!)

Just yesterday Nikki sent me an e-mail picture of my favorite turkey drumsticks from "Strongbow Inn Restaurant," (in Valparaiso, Indiana). The picture featured the "Gobbler's Delight," with the biggest drumsticks that you will ever see on a dinner plate. Only Nikki! She knew it would make me smile, and sure enough, it did. In fact, that was her main concern when she heard that I had been diagnosed. Her question was, "What T.V. show or movie makes you laugh or feel good?" Being a psychologist herself, Nikki knew the research on the healing properties of laughter, (see "Anatomy of an Illness" written by Norman Cousins in 1979, and *Proverbs 17:22, DBY,* "A joyful heart promoteth healing; but a broken spirit drieth up the bones."). She determined that we would take advantage of this wisdom. She subsequently sent me several videos with "Frasier" and "Star Trek Next Generation," (with the hilariously flamboyant character, "Q"), and a book of jokes to boot!

Entry 38
Home group

One of the most dramatic reactions to our announcement came at a home group that Mark and I were facilitating. We were presenting the DVD series by Emerson Eggerichs called, "Love and Respect." The series is designed for married couples, and outlines biblical principles for a successful marriage. The foundation of the series stems from the scripture, *Ephesians 5:33*, "However, each one of you also must love his wife as he loves himself, and the wife must respect her husband."

We had just started the DVD series the week before, and had about 22 people crammed into our fairly small front room, sitting on everything from kitchen chairs to stools and folding lawn chairs. As we faced the group that evening, we felt awkward about sharing my diagnosis, yet we knew that these people would need to know. The plan was to take 16 weeks to slowly digest the DVD information, sharing our struggles and victories while making improvements in our marriages. This cancer stuff just might throw a wrench into our arrangement.

As we told this precious group of people our situation, you could have heard a pin drop onto our carpeted floor. There was a moment of regret that we had shared too much of our too immediate pain with a newly forming group of human beings and their natural tendencies toward shock and disassociation. It was only a moment…and then we knew. God had purposely placed these precious believers into our home "for such a time as this." (The concept is taken from the scripture, *Ester 4:14b*, "And who knows but that you have come to your royal position for such a time as this?")

They almost stumbled over each other in their rush to surround us, lay hands upon us, and fervently pray. They prayed for everything from peace and comfort to direct healing, claiming on our behalf, the scriptures that had been given to us, "No weapon formed against you shall prosper," (*Isaiah 54:17, NKJV*), and "And we know that in all things God works for the good of those who love him, who have been called according to his purpose." (*Romans 8:28*).

Whew! What *power* there is in the body of Christ when they come together, united in purpose, and fueled by God's word! Nobody was scared off by our announcement that night. We fluctuated between 12 and 25 people throughout the 16 weeks. I think that was pretty amazing, and I thank God for his perfect plan of involving us in these people's lives at exactly the right time. In fact, the DVD series is now regularly offered by an incredible couple who first viewed "Love and Respect" in our home. Tim and Lynn Mira celebrated 25 years of marriage this year, and as a gift to the Kauai community, they decided to make presenting the series one of their *many* ministries. (And the ripple effect of the waves of hope continues on…)

Entry 39
Client reactions

I was dreading telling my clients that I was diagnosed with breast cancer. It turned out to be a necessary evil that God used very powerfully in my life, and I believe, also in theirs. Most of the precious ones that God had guided through the doors of my psychological practice experienced an emotional reaction that lead them into tears of sadness, pain and identification. (There is a universal suffering that I find most are drawn into when cancer is involved.) All of them eventually turned to prayer, regardless of their level of faith. Each of those clients ended up at the foot of the cross, pleading with the Lord for my healing. There were those who did this in session, and those who later relayed to me their personal process of coming to terms with this cancer thing. I was completely dumfounded. God used my diagnosis to pull those people closer to him. How astoundingly creative! What a confounding of Satan's plan *that* must have been!

Naturally, I referred the majority of my clients to other psychologists for continued care. A few were at the end of their treatment and their cases were closed over the ensuing weeks. I did keep a couple of clients that I believed would actually benefit from walking through the treatment process with me. Post-hoc, I know with the Lord's leading, this decision was correct. It was during this time of uncertainty and turmoil that they learned to rely on God more profoundly than would have been possible otherwise. Additionally, they were given the opportunity to contribute to my victory over cancer, something that most definitely was a benefit for them as well as for me.

I had experiences with my long-time clients that are very close to my heart. Everyone found a unique way to express their support and connect with me through this period of time. I received a myriad of gifts. Just to name a few; there were homemade items like a gorgeous, scripture-embroidered purse, a lovely blanket and a handmade pillowcase. There were pink cancer symbols on everything from little pins to sticky notes, bookmarks, and jewelry. I was presented with vitamin supplements, books and DVD's on immune system enhancements, prayers, faith healings, and treatments. It was a wonderful way that clients demonstrated their loving support, and it brought our therapeutic relationships into a higher dimension of connection and trust...Satan was foiled again!

Entry 40
The Dr. Lam experience

I have a few friends from Bible study who battled cancer using non-traditional methods. It is interesting how God surrounded me with people who elicited help from an 86 year old Chinese medical doctor practicing on Oahu. His name is Dr. Frederick Lam. Let me tell you about our experience with Dr. Lam.

When Mark and I entered Dr. Lam's office, things seemed fairly normal. We were asked to sit in his waiting area. Even though there was really nothing unusual about this we were already on the alert for the abnormal. I had received an e-mail tipping me off, entitled, "No pink!" The e-mail, from one of my friends and fellow cancer survivors, warned me that I needed to be certain of something. She said that when I went to see Dr. Lam, I must remove all pink nail polish, wipe clean all pink lipstick, and for heaven's sake, do not wear any pink clothes! Nobody could adequately explain the reason for this, so I just complied thinking that explanation would come from the doctor himself.

We went into Dr. Lam's office together, and met his assistant, Arnoldo. After introductions I was asked to sit in a chair facing Dr. Lam, while Mark and Arnoldo observed. Dr. Lam asked me to hold a metal rod that he had wrapped with a wet towel. As I held the rod, Dr. Lam took my opposite hand and began placing an electrical probe on each of my fingers. He poked the sides of my fingernails on each hand, and then proceeded to do the same with each toenail. Accompanying each poking was a high pitched noise, something like a siren going off. The noise remained at a high pitch only briefly, and then died back down. There was no explanation of what in the world was going on, nor was there any recognition that this was the least bit peculiar. Mark and I kept glancing at each other with wide-eyed astonishment. Oh yes, before we began this "interesting" process, my purse was banned from the immediate area, due to its partial pink décor.

As Dr. Lam finished his initial assessment, he began to open drawers containing hundreds of glass receptacles. Each receptacle was labeled with its contents. Dr. Lam studied the results of the poking test that appeared on a computer screen and then selected what he determined to be the "appropriate" receptacles. Placing these lucky glass vessels into my hands, he resumed the poking procedure. Dr. Lam continued poking and watching the computer until he appeared satisfied with the resulting noises.

By this time, Mark and I were chomping at the bit to ask questions regarding this unorthodox method of diagnosing, and presumably treating, cancer. We were patiently told that this method had been used originally in eastern medicine. Dr. Lam and Arnoldo explained that the containers had actual pathologies, (viruses, cancers, diseases, etc.) inside them…now isn't that "special"?! They called the method of diagnosis, "electro-acupuncture" and the treatment, "mesenchymal reactivation using homeopathic nosodes." Now that calmed our nerves and answered all our questions completely! (Ha-Ha!!)

I believe that after two hours, Mark and I were more confused than we had been upon entering the office. But, we had a decision to make. Did we want to go ahead with the treatment? The chemicals, or nosodes, needed to be ordered from Germany, and could take over a month to receive. In the meantime, I would be injected with the initial nosodes, and we would empty our pocketbooks.

Once again, my faith-filled husband spoke in truth soaked, clear headed fashion, reminding me that we were not there to critique Dr. Lam's methods, but to gain benefit from them. He jogged my memory as to how we ended up in the good doctor's office. Mark reminded me that we had believed that God was leading us in this direction, regardless of how it "looked" in the natural. I crumbled under this wisdom, allowing myself to fork out the dough, although I gotta tell you, every Jewish and Irish bone in my body was aching from it!

Then I received my first nosode treatment injection, and was essentially told to drown myself in water over the succeeding 24 hours...or pay the price! As I discovered, the price was quite high. It included nausea, headaches and an incredibly irritating *over*-perception of strong odors.

Additionally I was warned to stay clear of sugar of *any* kind. That included the obvious candies and sweets, but much to my dismay, also included fruit, white rice, white flour, honey and anything else that could be used by the cancer cells to fortify themselves. One of my friends and fellow Dr. Lam groupies explained it this way. She asked me if I was familiar with the PET, (Positron Emission Tomography), scan commonly used to identify cancer cells. Then she reminded me that the solution patients drink prior to the scan is radioactive glucose...*sugar*. The sugar is quickly grabbed by the cancer cells, prompting the activity that is identified on the PET scan. That was good enough for me. No sugar in any form. Not while I still had active cancer cells in my body.

You can look for yourself at the research supporting this type of treatment, I know I did. It's there in the literature, hidden in back alley laboratories and non-traditional medical journals. All I can say about it at this point is that I have never felt as good as when I finished my 10 week round of injections.

By the way, the pink...well, I am still uncertain about this, but I will tell you the facts. When Dr. Lam gave me something pink to look at while he assumed the poking position, the sirens went off like crazy, indicating that this color dramatically affected my electrical-chemical reactivity. Dr. Lam likened it to being exposed to nuclear radioactivity. I conveyed this experience to my nuclear chemist father, and he hesitated a moment before commenting. He said, "Well… there *is* something different about the color pink…but I would like to talk to the doctor about it more." He hasn't had the opportunity, and I avoid most pink, even today. In addition, I remain on a low sugar diet because *I know* what my body likes to do with excess sugar!

Entry 41
East vs. West

As Mark and I shared our eastern medicine approach to cancer treatment with our scientifically minded families and friends, we received a *lot* of resistance. It was just the beginning of what would progress into an all-out *war* between our eastern and western medical practitioners. It is beyond my comprehension that in today's world, with all the complexities of creation becoming increasingly exposed by new technologies, we can even begin to think that taking one approach to treatment of any kind, will adequately address the intricacies of life and of the healing process. By taking a combined approach, Mark and I invited the battle between the diverse perspectives into our lives. Prior to my lumpectomy surgery I was faced with the first of many complicated decisions that would affect me for the rest of my life.

My western medical practitioners told me in no uncertain terms that I needed to have a "sentinel lymph node resection." They also told me that after the operation, I might experience problems with that arm. In fact, they warned me that I would have to live for the remainder of my life with the threat of developing, "lymphedema." Lymphedema occurs when fluid is retained and creates a swelling of the arm, due to problems within the lymphatic system. Symptoms may include; fatigue, a heavy swollen arm, skin discoloration and elephantiasis.

The prospect of developing lymphedema was quite sufficient to cause me to question whether the lymph node resection was truly necessary. My eastern medical practitioners
assured me that they would be treating the cancer directly,
and that "butchering my arm by taking the lymph nodes"
would be unnecessary. Dr. Lam indicated that he would
prefer I wait for any surgery until his nosode treatments were
completed. On the other end of the treatment continuum, my
western medical practitioners told me that if I were to wait
on surgery, or to eliminate the lymph node resection, I would
be setting myself up for the spread of cancer throughout my
body.

Mark and I did a lot of praying during our decision-
making process. We also gathered as much information as
we could from people we trusted. Our primary reliance was
on the Lord via claiming the scripture:

Isaiah 30:20-22, "Although the Lord gives you the bread
of adversity and the water of affliction, your teachers will
be hidden no more; with your own eyes you will see them.
Whether you turn to the right or to the left, your ears will
hear a voice behind you, saying, "This is the way; walk
in it."

We believed after careful consideration, that we should
go ahead with the lumpectomy and the sentinel lymph node
resection as the western medical practitioners had recommended. We also decided to continue with the eastern medical nosode treatments.

Entry 42
Battle with fear

Before my first surgery, there was a battle going on inside
my head. The battle was with fear. I suppose this is a normal

reaction to the cancer diagnosis, but one that is seldom discussed among Christians. Maybe it is because fear is known to be from the evil one, and there is shame attached to the fact that sometimes, it consumes us. After all, the Bible says about 366 times, "Do not fear," once for each day of the year!

Yet there was one night when I laid awake ruminating about my condition. It was like God was allowing me to cognitively rehearse each and every horrific possibility that I could conjure up. I thought about what my life would be like if I had to live with a ballooned arm, (lymphedema). I rehearsed how my body would likely respond to chemotherapy, and how sick I would be. I thought about every nuance and permutation of the disease including the big one, "What if I slowly, gradually deteriorated, and every penny of my family and extended family's finances were drained, and Kauai Bible Church was burdened with fund raising to pay my medical expenses, and Mark had to visit me, incapacitated in the hospital for months or even years before I finally was taken to heaven?!" There, I said it. *That* was the biggest fear. It was the "hanging on" stuff and its effect on my dear husband, family and friends.

God allowed this to go on repeatedly throughout the night, the anxiety building with each additional tragic thought. Then, as I prayed for relief, the Lord impressed on me a question. "Which option would you choose?"

He showed me the ramifications of my choice in two different scenarios. In the first one he took me home without delay. There was minimal suffering and trauma involved. When I arrived in heaven, there were many people who were affected by my life, lined up to thank me and tell me how my faith influenced them to pursue salvation in Jesus.

In the second scenario I experienced much suffering. All of my deepest fears were realized, (it was a slow, costly, horrendous process of dying), and then I was taken home to the

Lord. In heaven there was a lineup again, but this time it was so long that it seemed to have no end. There were so many lives affected by my journey through cancer, that I could not count them.

Even as I type this, I have feelings that I cannot label. These emotions are partially related to pain, but mostly related to thankfulness and awe that God could use me as a vehicle for saving souls. After the visions, my choice was so simple. I chose more. More Lord. Use me for your purposes and your glory. Bring more into your Kingdom.

It was also a "Job," (from the Bible), lesson for me. Who am I to tell God how my life should unfold? He needed no direction from me, but what he did ask was that I trust him to make the right decision. Once I recognized this and truly accepted his sovereignty over my life, *I was free!*

A peace settled over me that night and it has never left me. It is peace that surpasses all understanding. The peace of God is not dependent on any diagnosis or trial. I chose to live in that freedom, trusting God completely.

Entry 43
Mark Willman

I have been trying to move forward on this journal since we came back from a ten-day visit with my family in Oregon, and each direction has been a dead end. I keep typing and then deleting. Just now, I prayed for the Lord to lead me, and as usual, he has answered my plea. It is time for me to give you some insight into my gift from God, my best friend, my "soul mate" and lover, Mark Willman.

I met Mark at a computer class during my final year at Purdue University. The class was an introduction to the Purdue computer system, something that I was determined to master well enough to perform my own statistical calculations for my dissertation. The night before the class I had been up half the night arguing with my soon-to-be ex-boy-friend, Bob. I arrived late and chose the only open seat that I noticed in a classroom of about 200. I just happened to sit right next to Mark.

During the hour-long class I proceeded to chomp on jelly beans, hoping to stay awake enough to encode some of the information presented. As I drifted off to sleep, the jelly beans that I was holding began to drop onto the floor, making a loud snapping sound. This sound was just loud enough to alert me as I drifted off, prompting me to jerk my conscious-ness back into the classroom and my head to an upright and fully locked position of attentiveness. I believed this method of staying awake was working pretty well for me, and after class I bent down to pick up the stray "alarm-beans" that had fallen under my desk. As I finished picking up after myself I suddenly looked up to see a huge grin accentuated by a handle-bar mustache, coming from the man in the next seat. That beaming face was the face of my Mark.

Although he might say otherwise, I believe that it was "love at first sight." After a few minutes of exchanging information about ourselves, I knew I would see him again. Mark had made it…through a Ph.D. program that is. He had graduated from the University of Illinois with a Doctorate in Agronomy, and had secured a job as a "Post-Doc" at Purdue, working on corn and rice-breeding projects. I was genuinely impressed. I gave him my office number and told him that I had been at Purdue for five years, and could introduce him to some people if he was interested. (My primary motive was to further introduce him to *this* person!)

Two days later my office partner was bursting with the news that some "new man" had come to visit me. I knew it was Mark. He left his office number, and I decided to pay him a visit. That is how our relationship began.

There is a story we tell that is truly unbelievable within the context of Purdue University and its student population of over 50,000. After our final computer class, neither of us wanted to leave each other's company, so we decided that we would continue talking at a local establishment where there was music and dancing. I told Mark that I needed to go home first, to pick up some money, and he said ditto. He asked me where I lived, and then just stood there staring wide eyed in reaction to my reply. I said, "Where do you live?" And his answer left me dumbfounded. We apparently lived at the exact same address. I lived in the house and Mark lived in a remodeled garage, on the same property. As you can imagine, we had a lot to discuss after that!

You may say it's just coincidence, but we believe that without God's intervention of connecting us via the computer class, guiding us to sit right next to each other, we very well may have never met. Our schedules were so different, and the entrances to our places were facing opposite directions, separated by the yard. God truly arranged our lives for "such a time as that." (Reference the book of Esther.)

Although this cancer journal is not about our marriage, it really is. As I have shared earlier in this journal, we went through a *lot* in the 25 years that we have known each other, and even more in our 21 years of marriage. I will not repeat what has been shared via our testimony from the "Miracle on Molokai," but I will tell you that when God said he will join man and woman to become one, (*Genesis 2:24*, NKJV, "Therefore a man shall leave his father and mother and be joined to his wife, and they shall become one flesh.") he really means it. We fought against this reality over the course of our two and one half year separation, but the fact remained that when God promised to join us in marriage, he kept his end of the deal. As we returned to this foundation of truth, (that we had been joined as one), we have received the benefits that God provides to a faith-filled marriage. And for me, that included a husband who would carry the cross of cancer, each step of the journey, as if it were his own... because it was, and it still is.

Mark is a faithful, compassionate servant of the almighty Lord. Every day he grows closer to Jesus, and every day he becomes more Christ-like. I was so grateful when Kauai Bible Church honored him by voting him as a "Deacon," an honor that is perfect for this "servant-leader." Although it was not intended to be leaked out, it was somehow announced that Mark had been voted in *unanimously* by the church membership. (This result had never before been accomplished in the history of Kauai Bible Church.)

That's my Mark. Everybody loves him who knows him, and he truly loves them back. He is exceptional in that he also loves his enemies, those who do him harm. He takes the word of God seriously, doing his very best to live Jesus out loud. He says that he would die for me, and I believe him. I would die for him as well. We are one, together, and together, we fight the cancer battle, claiming and receiving the victory every day.

Entry 44
First surgery

I can *do* "front and center!" Most of my life I have been involved in performance arenas and I have evolved from a frightened little girl who at four years of age, refused to go on stage at a children's dance recital, into an adult personality who thrives in the spotlight. Although this particular spotlight is not one that I craved, I actually do feel comfortable being the one battling cancer. I have no doubt that God would give me the strength I would need to reverse roles if ever Mark needed me to be his care-giver, but I am fully aware that it would not be second nature to me.

Before my lumpectomy surgery I remember lying comfortably on the gurney awaiting my turn. I had carefully fixed my hair, put on my make up, and I must have been beaming with the excitement of being the object of so much attention. I say that because of a couple of comments that were made prior to being wheeled into the operating room.

One of the nurses stood at the foot of my bed slowly shaking his head. I asked him what he was thinking, and he said, "You just don't look sick." I immediately seized the opportunity to demonstrate my faith as I shouted, "I am *not* sick. I am healed by God's grace! Don't worry about me!" He looked a bit shocked, but did manage a smile. Then my illustrious surgeon, Dr. Emilia, came into the room. She began to explain the surgical procedures and then she stopped and said, "You look beautiful." I decided I was pleased that while I was out of commission, undergoing a slashing, I could at least look good. That's gotta be God's grace, don't you think?

Here is the e-mail we sent after surgery:

E-mail Post Surgery

Subject: Update on surgery
Date: Wed 05/21/08 11:00 PM

Dear family and friends:

It is surgery day, and we are home, happy and sending out this Victory message! After MUCH prayer, deliberation, consultation, etc. we decided to go for the "Lumpectomy." This morning we had the surgery, or rather, Val had the surgery, and Mark did the support and pacing-dance for about two hours. It went well, with preliminary tests showing no spread of the cancer into the lymph nodes. They did a "lymph node resection," taking only three nodes, as they identified the proper ones to take that would most likely illustrate any spreading. This identification procedure was done with radi-

ation injected into the skin, and then gamma ray pictures were obtained for this purpose. It was funny that seeing the signs warning of radioactivity actually made Val feel more comfortable, as it brought back associations with life in Richland, Washington growing up. Interesting how God uses all things for our good and his glory!

We returned home about 1:30pm. Val was a bit nauseous from the anesthesia for a few hours, but is feeling fine now. Only a bit of pain and fatigue from the ordeal. Val recalls talking with the Anesthesiologist several times, trying to weasel out of the anesthesia...to no avail. She thinks he must have turned up the volume a bit to put her out quick, as she was still trying to reason with him on the operating table. The next memory she has is waking up in recovery with several nurses looking over her.

The pathology report will take about one week to return from analysis. We are praying for a great report of miraculous healing, and are prepared for whatever the Lord has for us to address next. We will make any necessary decisions at that point.

We are also following a holistic treatment regimen by a famous Naturopathic Physician on Oahu, named Dr. Frederick Lam. He is an 86 year old Chinese man, and has "saved the life" of some of Val's clients and friends. People travel from all over the world to see him, and Val and Mark spent three hours with him and his assistant last Friday. He does something called, "Bio-Energetics." We are following his treatments, taking many natural supplements, and will continue seeing him until the cancer is GONE completely!! Val already feels better since beginning on Friday. (Val believes that this was something very similar to a treatment she was getting from Dr. Stephen Smith in Richland, for her allergies...and that really helped, but was cut short due to our move to Hawaii. We guess God desired us to pursue that treatment, as he hooked us up here to continue it for cancer as well as the allergies.)

Now to the great stuff...we attended the Samoan Fire Knife World Championships in Oahu. It was SPECTACULAR!!!! Val went Wednesday with her dear friend, Darlene, and they shopped and had a blast-and then got blasted by the fire dancers that evening. There were four girls, and about ten groups/duets. AWESOME!! Then Mark came on Thursday evening, and Mark and Val went to the competition on Friday and Saturday. We have no superlatives for how fantastic it was. The show at the Polynesian Cultural Center on Saturday, incorporating the finals of the Samoan Fire Championships, was as good a show as we have probably ever seen. We suggest you try to plan a trip to visit US, and while on Oahu, GO!!!

God is good...all the time. He is our great, merciful healer. We love him and all of you too. Thank you so much for all your prayers and love and compassion and generosity. We will continue to keep you all posted, unless you tell us to remove you from our list. We will love and respect you either way.

We gotta go have some dinner-it's getting late here. Thank you all, so very much.

Aloha Blessings and Lots of Love,

* Val and Mark...and Pumpkin!*

After my surgery we came home and I slept off the nausea caused by the anesthesia. Mark said he was a bit concerned, but I knew it would not last. Pastora Darlene at Kauai Bible Church had arranged for our meals to be cooked and delivered by precious members of the congregation. Each meal was carefully prepared to adhere to my no-sugar regimen. By the day after surgery, I was answering the door feeling quite awkward about accepting help with cooking when I believed I was perfectly capable of doing it myself. In fact, a week post-surgery I attended the Kauai "Polynesian Festival" Samoan Fire Knife workshop…as a spectator, of course. I just wanted to watch. Mark came with me to be sure that observing was *all* that I would try to accomplish!

A funny side note about this part of the journey…the breast that had the "lumpectomy" swelled up to about three times my normal size! We joked about having the other one "pumped up" to match it.

Most of what I remember about that week involves attempting to get back to some type of "normalcy" as quickly as possible. Because the cancer diagnosis dictated immediate chaotic changes in lifestyle, any little part of my world that could partially reflect familiarity, helped me to regain stability and grasp onto the peace of God. I love the verse, *Philippians 4:6-7,* "Do not be anxious about anything, but in every situation, by prayer and petition, with thanksgiving, present your requests to God. And the peace of God, which transcends all understanding, will guard your hearts and your minds in Christ Jesus." I prayed it and claimed it a *lot* throughout my journey.

Entry 45
Victory over cancer fight continues

A week following my initial surgery we met with Dr. Emilia for the pathology report.

This is the e-mail we sent following our appointment:

Subject:
"Victory over cancer" fight continues (Val and Mark Willman)
Date: Thu 05/29/08 11:54 PM

Dear friends and family:

Sometimes there are just not good ways to begin, and this is one of those times. We did not receive "good" news today as we were presented with the cancer pathology report. The report indicated that Val has two forms of cancer, one in the form of the lump that was removed, and the other in a more invisible form that infiltrates the milk ducts of the breast. This was not identifiable by the previous tests, but was found in the analysis of the material that our doctor removed. Additionally, there was cancer identified in one of the three lymph nodes that were removed. This was also not discovered upon initial analysis performed the day of surgery.

God is good...all the time! *This is still true, and we are standing on this for stability as our adventure with "Victory over cancer" continues. (We have named you all the "Victory over cancer group" for e-mail updates!! Thank you for your prayers and love as we fight this battle together!)*

So, what does all this mean practically? We will need additional surgery to perform a mastectomy, (we believe this is the best option presented to us taking into consideration the new information about the cancers involved). At that time the doctor will also remove the identifiable lymph nodes. This operation will be performed during the same surgery, and the date is set for six days from today, Wednesday, May 4th at KVMH Hospital in Waimea, Kauai. Val will stay overnight and may return home the next day pending good progress. The healing process will be more extensive for these procedures. It is likely that she will be recuperating for 10-14 days. After this time, they will have more information about the nature of the spread of cancer, and more tests will be done to identify any other significant developments in Val's body. The next step will be chemotherapy. This can be done on Kauai, a Blessing in disguise!

*In the past whenever Val heard the word, "chemotherapy," the image of "last resort" generally came in close association. Val really thought that if she ever heard that SHE would need chemo, she would most likely have the graceful response of throwing up in the doctor's office! However, we thank God for his Grace and the Holy Spirit's presence. Today, when Val heard the word chemotherapy, she had none of the nausea, but what did come quickly to mind was..."Lance Armstrong!!!" Those of you, who are aware of Lance's battle and Victory over cancer, recognize the AWESOME power that is associated with his story. For those who are unaware, Lance is a Professional Cyclist, who is a seven-time winner of the famous, "Tour-de-France." He was diagnosed with extremely severe cancer in 1996, and fought through the treatments only to come out stronger, faster and more able than ever. His seven consecutive Tour wins were 1999-2005...post-cancer! Those yellow bracelets you may see on folks that say, "Live**strong**," are from Lance and his "Lance Armstrong Foundation," a leading support and research organization in the world of cancer treatment today. (Yes, Val will be getting a yellow bracelet!)*

We wish that we had better news to share with you, but we are confident in these things:

God is large and in charge!

We can do all things through Christ who strengthens us! **(Philippians 4:13)**

No weapon formed against us will prosper! **(Isaiah 54:17)**

He will use this too for his purpose and our good! **(Romans 8:28)**

We love you all and pray for double Blessings for you, as you continue blessing us by standing with us in this battle.

Val and Mark

I can still remember the initial shock and the sadness I experienced in Dr. Emilia's office that day as she informed us of the pathology report. This wasn't the way it was supposed to go according to my fairy-tale expectations. It was only a lump, and the lump was gone. There was nothing found in the lymph nodes upon initial examination, and that is usually correct…usually. And then, the "Why ME's?" came flooding into my mind followed closely by the still small voice in the recesses of my mind asking, "Why *not* me?" Fortunately, that is what came out of my mouth after initially crying and embracing my dear husband. I exclaimed, "The question is not, why us, but why *not* us?" Why not people of faith, like us, who could continue declaring the word of God as truth, regardless of a particular situation or diagnosis or prognosis!

The presence of the Holy Spirit was never more obvious to me as when Dr. Emilia began discussing the need for chemotherapy. Even typing the word, over a year post-hoc, forces my stomach to turn with disdain. I had literally practiced in my mind how I would react if I ever heard the word, chemotherapy, applied to me. That reaction involved immediate expulsion of not quite digested food. It never happened. I consider it a miracle. What *did* happen surprised the heck out of me. She said, "Chemotherapy…" I said, "Lance Armstrong!"

As the e-mail insinuates, by championing, both bicycling and cancer, Lance's story offered me a platform that I could firmly entrench myself on, declaring my cancer battle to be winnable! Identifying with his success gave me hope, as it has so very many cancer survivors. What is truly unique in my situation is the preparation that God did with me, for the very moment I would hear the word, chemotherapy, in the office that day.

When Mark and I lived in Indiana we had a friend who participated in triathlons. Dr. Paul Sommer, Podiatrist and friend, originally introduced us to Lance Armstrong and his unique physiology that had been transformed by his extraordinary battle with cancer. Paul had a poster of Lance in his office, and shared with us an enthusiasm for the sport, and for Lance. After moving to the State of Washington, Mark and I were introduced to the television coverage of the famed, "Tour de France," by my parents. We have been following the Tour, and Lance's career, ever since. I really believe that God orchestrated these events and nurtured our affinity for Lance's story, for "such a time as this." (Again, I refer to the book of Esther, and I emphasize the redundancy as illustration of God's complete involvement throughout our lives.) If God knows the number of hairs that are on my head, (*Matthew 10:30*), how could he *not* know exactly what was required to be ready for that moment in Dr. Emilia's office?

So...I didn't throw up. What I *did* do is proceed to call the "troops" into battle. Mark and I made the calls, we sent the e-mail and we dug deep into prayer. By this time, our wise and determined Pastor, Merv Walker, exclaimed that we, (Kauai Bible Church), had taken *enough*! He declared a three-day fast and prayer, calling the entire church to come together for three nights prior to my surgery, to pray together. He urged those who could not be present to fast and pray on their own. During that time we brought before the Lord not only my needs, but those of many in our church who had been affected by health concerns and a variety of debilitating events that truly seemed like spiritual attacks. Our church's efforts were joined by many, including my parents, friends and even neighboring churches. It seemed like I was being added daily to additional prayer lists. There were churches in my hometown of Richland, Washington that placed me before the Lord. We were put on most every church prayer list from those Christians on our 85 member "Victory over cancer list," (representing places around the world). Mark discovered that many of his co-workers at Pioneer Seed were joining in the praying. The most unusual list that we heard of was a Christian Motorcycle Association in California.

One day I received a call from a woman that had never met me. She told me that she was calling out of obedience to the Lord's urging. She had heard about my story from a Bible study group on the north shore of Kauai, and believed that she needed to relay a message from God. The message was simply, "Be encouraged. You are loved." That was it. I never heard from this woman again, and I have never met her since. It makes me wonder if she exists within the realm of humanity, or if she was an angel, sent to provide me with an emotional boost.

During the first of three "fast and pray" nights at Kauai Bible Church, we believe that I received my healing. Let me tell you how it unfolded.

Entry 46
The Healing

Pastor Merv requested everyone participate in the three day "fast and prayer." He encouraged us all to meet at the Church for one hour each night. Kauai Bible Church is a small, but very mighty Church, just recently voted as the "Best place to worship on Kauai." Our congregation population is about 200, with about half to three quarters attending the Sunday services.

At the first hour-long prayer meeting there were about 50 people. We began with prayer and guitar music played by our faithful and incredibly talented music Pastor, David Leong. It was during one of the songs that I had the impression I was supposed to get up from my seat and dance! I leaned over to tell Mark what I believed I was hearing from God, and he said, "Yes, get up and dance!" I had never done this before, but for some reason, I did not feel a bit awkward. I danced and spun, making movement with my hands and body to fit the lyrics. I remember the song too. Here it is:

"Mighty to Save," Hillsong

Everyone needs compassion
Love that's never failing
Let mercy fall on me
Everyone needs forgiveness
The kindness of a Saviour
The hope of nations
Saviour
He can move the mountains
My God is mighty to save
He is mighty to save
Forever
Author of salvation
He rose and conquered the grave
Jesus conquered the grave
So take me as You find me
All my fears and failures
Fill my life again
I give my life to follow
Everything I believe in

Now I surrender
Shine your light and let the whole world see
We're singing
For the glory of the risen King — Jesus

(Permission to reprint lyrics granted by Jay Winter, Licensing Administrator, EMI CMG Publishing)

As I type this I had *no idea* that I remembered what the song actually was. It is very clear to me that the Lord desired that I share the exact song. I am crying tears of thankfulness as I listen to a version of the song on U-Tube while typing this into the journal. I remember it like it was yesterday. I remember the joy that I felt as I danced. It was perfect. It was true. Jesus conquered the grave, and he would conquer my cancer. I danced, surrendered, and trusted God...and I shined my light, the light of Jesus.

Pastora Darlene later said that it was very apparent to her when the healing came, it was during the dance. I believe it.

Then there was prayer like I have never experienced before. Pastor Merv suggested the ladies "lay hands on Val and pray for her." Again, the scene is vivid in my mind. More than twenty beautiful, compassionate ladies of God, just floating across the room toward me. There was laughter and lifting of prayer. We all claimed the victory that had just been imparted to me during my dance, shouting "We claim *V-I-C-T-O-R-Y!*"

Entry 47
Second surgery decisions

Upon examination of the pathology report, Dr. Emilia gave us a couple of options for treatment. She said that she would do one more lumpectomy, in an attempt to save what remained of my breast, or she could perform a mastectomy.

In addition to this surgery, she stated that she would be taking the remaining lymph nodes. (Specifically, levels one and two.) She was very firm about this due to the discovery of a small piece of cancer in one of the sentinel nodes.

I sent my pathology report to Dr. Lam, requesting any recommendation he might have for us. No reply. His opinion had not changed and he saw no need to reiterate it.

Again, Mark and I had to look to the Lord for direction. We realized at this point that our marriage retreat that had been scheduled at the Kauai Marriott Resort would have to be postponed. This postponement was actually more difficult for us than the surgery decisions. (We were very grateful to the Marriott for refunding our down payment and allowing us to renege on our contractual obligations.)

This treatment decision was one that I realized needed to come from me. Nobody wanted to be responsible for taking my breast, and I can't blame them. For me this was a "no brainer." Whack the diseased thing off! When my dad heard that I would be undergoing a mastectomy, his response made me laugh. "Now Val, this will be nothing more than a minor shark bite!" (This was perfectly apropos for someone living in the Hawaiian Islands!)

Many people have sensitively asked me if it is difficult adapting to life as a woman who has only one breast. The truth is that I have never looked back. Maybe it is related to the fact that I am pretty dinky anyway, or that I never had children, so a maternal nurturing association was never formed. Mark seems OK with it, telling people that he "kinda misses ol' lefty!" More likely it is related to my identity as a baton twirler. Yes, you read it correctly. Let me explain myself.

If you told me that I needed the fingers of my left hand taken off, I would most likely be devastated. It has been those "gifted" fingers that have contributed to who I am as a champion, as a winner and more than that, to who I am in the Lord. I see my baton twirling as a special blessing from God. It has allowed me to share the experiences I have had in a very unique way, consistent again, with who I am. The idea that I would no longer be able to spin the baton and share my related testimony makes my heart very heavy. But it wasn't my fingers…and just maybe I have been freed up via the removal of my left breast, to move and spin a bit more quickly!? (There is always a silver lining if you look closely enough.)

Entry 48
Surgery two

Subject: Val's June 4 surgery - "A blessed success!"
Date: Wed 06/04/08 11:40 PM

Everyone,

I (Mark) am writing an update for Val as she rests from her surgery in Kaua`i Veterans Memorial Hospital (KVMH) in Waimea. The surgery was a success - thank you, Lord! Thank you all for your prayer, concern, and love. We both appreciate it and know if it wasn't for your support, the success would not have happened. We are overwhelmed with God's grace expressed in the success and in your love!

We arrived at the hospital at 7am and they had Val on an IV by ~8:30am. They did not roll her into the O.R. until 1:30pm since they had nine surgeries that day. In the waiting time, we talked, prayed, read the Bible and sang songs with the help of my beginners' ukulele strumming, along with Pastor Merv and his wife Darlene. I got a call from the doctor at ~3pm saying they had removed the left breast, took out a cluster of lymph nodes, with only having to use 1 drain tube, and put a port on the right side for subsequent chemotherapy. Val was returned to her single occupancy double room awake, (they wanted to put another female in the room but housecleaning had forgotten to replace the dividing curtain), not feeling nausea, and hungry! She ate a chef salad and soup and is resting nicely. I will return to spend the night with her on a chair that folds out into a "cot."

We expect the doctor to release her tomorrow morning. She will not be able to drive for 10-14 days. She has cancelled her clients and we have postponed the Marriage Retreat scheduled for June 20-21. During the recovery time, we expect to get the pathology report and chemotherapy recommendations. I will balance (with your help) taking care of Val, myself, and my job.
Thank you again for your support in all the ways God directs and has gifted you. Please continue to pray for a clean report with minimal chemotherapy - that this cancer in her has not prospered and is eliminated - and for a rapid and healthy recovery.

We love you all.

God bless,

Mark & Val

That night was a much more pleasant one than the one after my first surgery. The more experienced anesthesiologist had made some adjustments to my surgical doses and I did not have any nausea! It was wonderful, and so my appetite returned as soon as my head cleared.

I was prepared to wake up with two clumsy tubes hanging off me for drainage purposes, but because of my tiny size, (here's that silver lining again), I needed only one. My doctor required that I remain hospitalized over-night for monitoring purposes, and so Mark pulled up a cot and stayed by my side. He endured the torture of constant interruptions in sleep throughout the night, and when we went home the next day, I believe he was more tired than I was!

Entry 49
Surgical success: lymphedema fears

When we left the hospital it was a bright, sunny day in Waimea, Kauai. We took advantage of it as you will read in the next e-mail we sent out:

Subject: Continuing to Claim Victory! (Written by Val)
Date: Fri 06/06/08 07:59 PM

Dear Victory over cancer Group:

*"This is the day that the Lord has made. I will rejoice and be glad in it!" (From **Psalm 118:24, NKJV**)*

I AM rejoicing and I AM glad today, as I feel the effects of your prayers and love. Thank you all, SO very much! I am healing nicely, up and about doing a little of this and that around the house. Yesterday, yes, the day after surgery, I was discharged at 9am. Mark and I took off in the car for a tour of the far West side of Kauai, stopping to admire the Waimea town overlook, visiting the pier, and then snagging a huge "shaved ice" (Hawaiian snow cone) at JoJo's, where they had the sugar free variety, just for ME!! (Gotta keep up my anti-cancer diet of NO sugar!) We had a wonderful meal that Mark made for lunch, and then rested. In the eve, after eating the fantastic dinner that one of our dear Church ladies brought for us, we walked around our block watching the sun set and chatted with neighbors. It was a miracle for sure!!!

I want to share a couple of things that God did with your efforts of prayer and support. First, it was quite the wait prior to surgery. We reported for duty at 7am, got hooked up to the IV-Buddy at 8am, and then waited until 1:30pm for my turn in surgery! We sang to the playing of Mark's ukulele, prayed, then talked and laughed, and waited. Then we sang some more, prayed for ALL the surgeries, talked, laughed, and waited...then we sang some more, prayed for the doctors, asked God to give YOU ALL double portions of the love and support that you were sending us, laughed and waited. There were many who were touched by the song and prayer as we roamed the hospital, tugging along the IV-buddy. At one time it seemed that the IV line was long enough for a bit of jump-rope, so we tried that too! At one point, I (Val) was doing a "mock-church" for fun, in the room, and decided to take it down the hallway..."This ought to get me in real quick!" was my comment...and we laughed. We didn't really go down the hallway, just making threats and having fun. Anyway, we had patience, and that was part of a miracle at work. (Take a bow for your part in this!)

Then I was wheeled into surgery. They asked the traditional questions for verification and security; along with, "Alright Val, what are we going to do with you today?" To which I replied, "My dad says that what you are going to do will be nothing more than a minor shark bite!" and noticing a lovely poster of "Sharks of the Pacific" they had on the wall entering the surgery room, I also said, "I notice you have their profiles up on your wall!" Everyone laughed, and I then recited the litany of events that would be taking place while I rested peacefully under God's control.

Another miracle...they adjusted the anesthesia, and I did NOT get sick at all! It was SUCH a Blessing. One of the anesthesiologists came to check on me the next day, asking if I woke up at all during surgery. My answer was nope, and he then asked me if I had questions for him. I said, "Did you FEEL the presence of God?" and he answered, "Well... everything went so PERFECTLY, it HAD to be God!" (Take a bow again; God IS responding to the prayers of all of you.)

Then, one of the best gifts that we received besides the successful surgery...when our Doctor came to check me out in the morning, she asked if she and her husband could still come to our Marriage Retreat! Our response included the postponement, but a resounding YES...and we will love to have them included when God allows the rescheduling of the Retreat! (It WILL be bigger and better than it ever could have been. The Lord has a more perfect plan. We have already begun to pray for those who God will be preparing to attend.)

*Now, something that I want to offer to all of you. This is the background: One of our wonderful church members gave us a card with some money inside, offering us love and support during this season of our lives. What is extraordinary about this is that the situation of this dear lady is very much like that of the "poor widow" in **Mark: 12** and **Luke: 21**. We knew we must do something special with this money. Remember my vow to get ahold of the Lance Armstrong bracelets? Well... they are ordered! We should be receiving them any day, and when we do, we would love to send you one as a representation of solidarity in this Victory over cancer battle. Please let us know if you would like to have one and send us your address. We will get them into the mail as soon as they arrive. My understanding is that it is customary to write the names of those affected by cancer with whom you are standing firm with in the battle, on the inside of the bracelet. We will be letting you know what we do with our bracelets, and we* *encourage you to do whatever is meaningful for YOU-with yours!*

*I want to thank you all again, for the prayers, love and support. You are ALL important to me in this battle. I am NOT in fear...actually; I am in AWE of what the Lord continues to do in my life and in the lives of those who are being affected by this journey/battle. I just got off the phone with someone I only met once, a couple years ago at a conference. She had heard about the postponement of the Marriage Retreat, and had a "Word of Knowledge" for me from God. The word included the powerful truth, "weeping may stay for the night, but rejoicing comes in the morning." (**Psalm 30:5**) It is spiritual morning here and we are so grateful.*

Let us hear from you, with your address, if you would like a bracelet. Otherwise, we will keep you posted unless you tell us to remove you from our list.

We love and appreciate you all so very much.

* Val and Mark *

The drain was clumsy, but manageable. Each time we dumped the accumulated liquid we dutifully recorded the amount and the time of elimination. (Dr. Emilia had requested we keep track so she could monitor the progress.) Mark helped me with it until I decided that I was capable of doing it myself. I guess I had a pretty good system of dissociation employed because I can't recall feeling anything except a mild irritation with all the documentation.

What I do remember concerns developing a pre-phobic reactivity in relation to my arm.

I sustained the typical nerve damage occurring as a result of the lymph node resection. Due to the many warnings I received about lymphedema, I had a hyper-sensitive focus regarding any sensation originating in the upper left quadrant of my body. Any little twinge of pain or anything rubbing up against my arm could set off an internal panic. The accompanying squirt of adrenalin would send me scampering into the bathroom to examine my arm for signs of excessive swelling. This excessive attentiveness to my arm drove me crazy! Even though I was informed that development of lymphedema in someone who was as athletic as myself was highly unlikely, I still experienced the internal battle with fear and doubt.

A few days post-surgery I decided to get outside into the Kauai sunshine by going for a walk. I soaked my arm in sunscreen. I also kept vigilant for any protruding bushes that might scrape my arm or bugs that could bite me. That first time I went on a walk, I was consumed with thoughts of over-exertion leading to obstructed circulation, escorting in arm ballooning.

Remnants of this emotion driven arm monitoring process still haunt me today. What I have learned is that there is a big fat *lie* embedded in the midst of the chaotic thoughts that lead to emotional upheaval and eventual physiological consequence. It is a sly ruse Satan has employed to distract me from God's truth about my situation. The lie is that God isn't enough. At the root of the fear of lymphedema are thoughts such as, "God isn't in control", "He won't prevent complications from occurring," or "He doesn't have time for little things like this."

The truth is that God knows me and my needs better than I do. He is perfectly capable of handling issues related to my arm and every other part of me. He is also the Master Healer, and can provide my arm with complete restoration. In addition, he will not allow anything that he does not use for my good and his glory! I have discovered that recognizing the lies and replacing them with thoughts based on truth keeps me out of panic mode. It can actually give me a method for gaining peace!

In psychology, the technique is called, "cognitive thought stopping." In the Bible, it is related to scriptures about taking captive thoughts that are not of God, (*2 Corinthians 10:5*, "We demolish arguments and every pretension that sets itself up against the knowledge of God, and we take captive every thought to make it obedient to Christ."). It is also consistent with another key scripture, (*Philippians 4:8*, "Finally, brothers and sisters, whatever is true, whatever is noble, whatever is right, whatever is pure, whatever is lovely, whatever is admirable—if anything is excellent or praiseworthy—think about such things."). Since I teach this technique to most every client I have ever worked with, maybe it is a good idea to practice it *myself!*

Entry 50
Second pathology report: the three

A week after my second surgery Mark and I cautiously entered Dr. Emilia's office to receive feedback from the pathology report:

Subject:
What a Miracle! (GREAT pathology report: Val and Mark)
Date: Fri 06/13/08 12:49 AM

Everyone!!

We are CELEBRATING the success of your prayers...the pathology report was excellent. Every last "indicator" that possibly could be good...WAS! There is NO indication of cancer remaining, there was NO cancer found in any other lymph node, (out of 22!), and there is a change in the activity of abnormal cells from a moderate to a LOW rating. There

148

is more technical info, but suffice it to say, we are claiming VICTORY and praising God for this MIRACLE. Please, do, take a bow for your efforts in prayer and loving support on our behalf.

We love you all and rejoice in what God continues to do with this experience.

* Val and Mark *

When Dr. Emilia gave us our results that day, we were prepared for whatever she would say. At least we thought we were. It was a good kind of shock when she told us that the pathology report came back completely clean. Even though we knew that God would heal me, I am not sure we thought it would happen so dramatically and quickly! We were just beginning to celebrate and claim our victory when our doctor's blatant comment sobered us up. She told us that in the past week she had to give three women in similar situations to me, dire pathology reports. One of them was a very good friend of hers.

Our demeanor immediately switched from celebration to sadness. For me, there was almost an element of guilt for being the one who God chose to heal. The phrase, "there but for the grace of God go I," seeped into my consciousness. I had questions that would not be answered over the course of my journey through cancer. The obvious mystery of how one person with persistent, even righteous faith is not graced with merciful healing yet another is, loomed confusingly at the forefront of my perception.

Mark says that in heaven he will have a flat forehead. The Bible tells us that it is in heaven with the Lord where we will understand completely, (*1 Corinthians 13:12, TNIV,* "For now we see only a reflection as in a mirror; then we shall see face to face. Now I know in part; then I shall know fully, even as I am fully known."). Mark says he will be slapping his forehead with the heel of his palm exclaiming, "Oh, that's why you allowed that to happen!" and, "Oh, now I understand *that!*" But until we get there, we are left to wonder, to question, to writhe in the anguish of attempting to use our puny little brains to conceptualize something that only God can fully enlighten us about. Or…we can just trust God.

We chose to trust God, releasing any guilt or shame of being the ones graced with his wonderful healing mercy. I believe as we did that, it freed us up to participate in God's plan more fully. We immediately determined that we would involve our "Victory over cancer" list in prayer for the three women our doctor told us about. We encouraged our supporters to pray for the "three" as well as anyone affected by cancer.

Entry 51
Continued treatment process

In the meantime, we were told that our voyage was just beginning. Dr. Amelia set up several appointments for us, and we proceeded to march forward, claiming our victory over each constituent of the process.

Our first appointment occurred six days later. It was a God ordained meeting with a well-intentioned oncologist. The reason I describe it so unenthusiastically will become clear as I outline our interactions.

I had prepared for this appointment by copying all the information I could find on the treatments that Dr. Lam was giving me. I also brought data pertaining to the supplements Dr. Lam and my dad had me taking, as well as other records about myself, my lifestyle and the changes I was making to combat further cancer developments. When the oncologist entered the room, it became immediately apparent that my file had not been read prior to entering the room. (I will henceforth refer to this oncologist as "Dr.O.")

Dr. O almost immediately spouted a recommendation to undergo radiation treatment on my breast prior to chemotherapy. We asked Dr. O which breast was being referred to, as I only had one remaining, and it had not been identified with any tumors. Dr. O then began flipping through my file, desperately searching for significant pieces of information. As Dr. O read parts of the file, more inappropriate recommendations were announced and then altered as Dr. O gained additional insight into my particular case.

As Dr. O became versed in my case, I offered the copies of materials I had brought in with me. This prompted the doctor's swift retreat behind an examining table and a stern tone of voice announcing that Dr. O believed there was no validity to any approach outside of mainstream Western medicine. Dr. O ultimately recommended a minimum of two rounds of hard core chemotherapy, to be followed by radiation treatment.

We were stunned. It was glaringly clear to us that this doctor had no intention of treating me as an individual case, nor did the doctor have any interest in understanding implications of the cancer treatment that I was already undergoing. Ironically, upon discovering that we were Christians, the doctor told us that we needed to "listen to that still small voice" as it would tell us what we should do. The implication here was that God would tell us that we needed to follow this doctor's leadership and pursue the recommended treatment. It is funny how God works. We did hear that voice, only it was *shouting* at us to get a second opinion.

Entry 52
LIVESTRONG Manifesto

My parents sent me the "LIVE**STRONG** Manifesto" during the course of my journey and I particularly appreciated the part about getting second, (or more), opinions:

The LIVE**STRONG** Manifesto
We believe in life.
Your life.
We believe in living every minute of it with every ounce of your being.
And that you must not let cancer take control of it.
We believe in energy: channeled and fierce.
We believe in focus: getting smart and living strong.
Unity is strength. Knowledge is power. Attitude is everything.
This is LIVE**STRONG**.
We kick in the moment you're diagnosed.
We help you accept the tears. Acknowledge the rage.
We believe in your right to live without pain.
We believe in information. Not pity.
And in straight, open talk about cancer.
With husbands, wives and partners. With kids, friends and neighbors. Your healthcare team. And the people you live with, work with, cry and laugh with.
This is no time to pull punches.
You're in the fight of your life.
We're about the hard stuff.
Like finding the nerve to ask for a second opinion.
And a third, or a fourth, if that's what it takes.
We're about preventing cancer. Finding it early. Getting smart about clinical trials.
And if it comes to it, being in control of how your life ends.
It's your life. You will have it your way.
We're about the practical stuff.

Planning for surviving. Banking your sperm. Preserving your fertility. Organizing your finances. Dealing with hospitals, specialists, insurance companies and employers.
It's knowing your rights.
It's your life.
Take no prisoners.
We're about the fight.
We're your advocate before policymakers. Your champion within the healthcare system. Your sponsor in the research labs.
And we know the fight never ends.
Cancer may leave your body, but it never leaves your life.
This is LIVE**STRONG**.
Founded and inspired by Lance Armstrong, one of the toughest cancer survivors on the planet.
(Reprinted with permission)

If you want to be emotionally moved, pull up this LIVESTRONG website and watch the touching video presentation and reading of the manifesto:

(http://www.live**strong**.org/Who-We-Are/Our-Strength/
LIVE**STRONG**-Manifesto)

Entry 53
Bone scan

The next day after our oncological fiasco I was scheduled to have a bone scan. The purpose was to determine if there were any indications of cancer spreading into my bones. Because a friend of mine had bone cancer, this scan took on a heightened level of apprehension for me. Although counter-intuitive, I felt more comfortable when I saw the radioactivity warning signs posted outside the Nuclear Medicine wing of Wilcox Hospital. Associations with my childhood experiences of life near the Hanford nuclear power plant in Richland, Washington flooded into my mind, coating my emotions with ironic familiarity that ultimately quelled my anxiety. I really do believe that God uses all things, and all experiences, to prepare us for what he allows into our lives.

The first thing I was told was that they were going to shoot me up with a "tracer" of radioactive substance, and it was going to hurt! The sweet-spirited technician told me that she would be right next to me, holding my hand, and that I had permission to squeeze as hard as I wanted, (this option offered akin to biting on a bullet). I thought to myself, "What on earth are they going to do to me?" And then, they injected the fluid. It stung, but wasn't nearly as bad as they lead me to believe. Then they booted me out of the hospital for about four hours, while the radioactivity had time to ooze throughout my system.

Upon my return, they sent me through a "whole-body scanner" that took its sweet time attempting to create a picture of any metabolic irregularities inside my bones. There was not much I could do at that point, except pray, and pray I did.

I really don't recall much else about the bone scan experience. I can tell you for certain that it isn't the scan so much as the kindness of that lovely technician that is most prominent in my memory banks. Amazing how cancer connects you with the most wonderful, caring people! It reminds me of Joseph from Scripture, when he told his brothers that what they meant for evil purposes, God used for good, (*Genesis 50:20*).

God will not be mocked. He says he will use all things for the good of those who love him, (*Romans 8:28*), and I believe that he will. Not just some things, but *all* things. I believe that God eventually turns every evil, even cancer, into a victory. In this case, God connected me with many beautiful people that I would have never met otherwise.

He used cancer, the unspeakably horrendous adversary of good, to provide a venue for blessing. Most cancer survivors concur with my experience.

Entry 54
Annelise's heart through hair

It was the weekend of our postponed marriage retreat, and my heart was feeling a bit low. In order to look presentable for our retreat, I had scheduled an appointment with my hairdresser to magically remove my "skunk line." (I fondly refer to my root outgrowth as a skunk line because of the contrast of the darker hair with the bleach blond.) Instead of getting prepared for the retreat, I was simply going in to get my hair done. What a letdown! Little did I know what was about to transpire...

Annelise Soderstrom is a lovely woman who truly cares about her clients. When she asks how you are doing, as she begins to comb through your hair, she really does want to know. That day I decided to let her into my world of concern, driven by my cancer diagnosis.

I thought it best to give her the chance to opt out of working with me, depending on how she felt about the possibility of chemotherapy and hair loss. "Of course I want to continue working with you," she said. And then she told me that her mother had battled breast cancer. Annelise said that her mom went through chemotherapy and lost her hair, but she won her battle and is now cancer free.

Then Annelise began to tell me all kinds of information that she had collected over the years of working with cancer clients. She even had the name of a local Kauai woman who sold wigs, and while we were waiting for my hair to magically change colors, Annelise called her.

I felt so much better knowing that just down the street I could pick up a hair style of my choosing! As I discussed the options with Annelise, I actually began to look forward to this process. Annelise assured me that whatever I chose, she would work with. We would walk through this together. Again, I was not alone. Cancer has a knack of connecting people, and this was just one more instance of a deepening relationship that I have treasured dearly along this journey.

Entry 55
Question

As we entered into the testing period, there was a question forming in the recesses of my mind. I decided to pose it to the "medical professionals" who were on our "Victory over cancer" list:

Subject: From Val: a question for my Medical Pro's
Date: 06/08

Victory Over cancer Medical Pro's:

I have a question for the Medical Professionals regarding a theory that I have for my one lymph node that read positive for cancer. I am uncertain if this is possible, and would value your opinions very much.

The description of the cancer that was located in Sentinel Lymph Node #3 was as follows: "Metastic ductal carcinoma, 3 mm, extending beyond capsule of lymph node" ...The original doctor that examined the sentinel lymph nodes and the tumor that was taken out in my first surgery, stated this, "No definitive lymphovascular invasion identified." It was my surgeon who called over to the Oahu lab and discussed this with another doctor, saying that if there was a piece of cancer discovered in the lymph node, then she believed that it was significant, and that the lymph node dissection was now necessary, along with chemotherapy. That second doctor agreed, and the second surgery was completed, revealing that there were NO additional nodes that had evidence of cancer in them. (Also, the original exam indicated no presence of cancer in the sentinel nodes, during surgery, which was the reason my surgeon did not do any further lymph node dissection at the time of the first surgery.)

My theory is as follows:

During the biopsy of the original tumor, the radiologist had a very difficult time removing pieces of the tumor. He indicated that it was the hardest tumor he had ever worked with. I was awake and not under any sedation, and I recall that the needle biopsy tool that he used took samples of approximately 3 mm, with "snipping sounds." There were more snips than samples taken out of my body. Is it possible that one of the snips of the original tumor traveled into the lymph node, and was found there upon original removal and examination? I ran this theory past my surgeon, and she said research has indicated that this does not happen. I understand where she may be coming from, and desire outside opinions before I let go of this theory. Is it even POSSIBLE? (With my very limited knowledge of how the body deals with cancer and other impurities that it finds in the system, it sounds logical, but is it even consistent with body operations?)

I will appreciate any input here. If you choose not to comment, that is fine as well...I just thought I would ask.

Blessings to you all!

* Val *

I don't know how far-fetched this theory sounds to you, but to me, it is entirely plausible. If you would've been where I was, experiencing the incredibly thorny procedure of repeatedly unsuccessful attempts at cutting a sample off my unusually tough tumor, you might have had the same ideas floating around your head.

I have to also tell you that it was only after several days of pondering my results that I had an "aha" moment. In this moment, I recognized that the size of the biopsy samples were listed as exactly the same size as the piece of cancer they located in my lymph node. Additionally, Dr. Lam had cautioned me about allowing the doctors to "fool around with my tumor" because he believed that spreading could occur during the biopsy process. As one of my cancer sur-viving, Dr. Lam following friends said, "Don't be alarmed if they discover evidence of cancer in the lymph nodes…that's where impurities are supposed to go!"

The answers I received varied widely from "*no-way,*" to "*well, unlikely, but maybe…*" I will say that my western medicine specialists were all in agreement that this would not happen. Because of the way it materialized in my mind, I still wonder if God didn't reveal it to me. In any event, it provided additional motivation for the research I performed that eventually lead down a different road for my answers.

Entry 56
Help from Dr. Sue

The following was extracted from a communiqué with my leg angioplasty doctor, Dr. James Wong:

To: Wong, James MD
Subject: From Val

Dear James:

I just wanted you to know how we went about trying to get a re-evaluation. First, we had a disturbing professional encounter with Dr. O. The doctor seemed very overwhelmed, over-extended and had not even looked at my reports prior to entering the room and making recommendations. (The first recommendation was for us to go get radiation on the breast that had already been removed...it went on like this for over an hour.)

Anyway, I indicated that we were interested in getting another view and there was no objection. My sister in law, an In-Vitro Fertilization specialist who practices in the Bay Area of California, contacted a cancer expert and got a recommendation from him for Dr. Cho's group on Oahu. I called for an appointment, but could not get in. My sister in law, Susan Willman, called and spoke directly with Dr. Yee. He agreed to see me on the Friday that we were already planning to go see Dr. Lam, (my Naturopathic, M.D.).

On the fun side, we are planning to turn the trip to Oahu to see Dr. Lam and Dr. Yee, into an anniversary jaunt! We will be on the Northshore for two days, attending something we discovered last visit..."Once-a- Month Church." This is a "church" service held at the Haleiwa park, and is geared to the homeless. They are unbelievable, giving away items via a "lottery," (from toilet paper and canned goods to candy for the children, and even automobiles!) They have a blast, all the while playing music, dancing, and praising God in any way imaginable. Their messages are simple and right on. If you can believe this, they don't take a monetary offering...

they GIVE one! Each person receives a two dollar bill. They emphasize that Jesus doesn't want your money, He wants YOU!

We were so impressed that we are staying for that "Once-a- Month" service, and then traveling over to Lanai, for our 18th wedding anniversary! We are planning to spend the week in Lanai, staying at the resort...something we NEVER do. It seems we usually try to pay as little as possible for our accommodations, knowing we won't be in the room much anyway. But we desired to do something really different for this anniversary. It is funny how the cancer diagnosis changes perspectives dramatically-for the better.

Dr. Susan Willman, my sister in law, took the reins and opened the door for me to get a second opinion from one of the most widely respected cancer treatment groups in our state. I was very thankful for her help due to the fact that I was getting nowhere with my efforts to secure an appointment. I do not believe it is any coincidence that Dr. Yee was the representative from the group who agreed to see me. (I will explain what I mean later in this journal.)

In addition, you notice the part of the e-mail about discovering the "Once-a-Month Church." Let me tell you how that connection unfolded:

Once-a-Month Church

During our May visit to Dr. Lam, Mark and I decided to stay on the north shore of Oahu. The north shore is known for its incredible surfing and beauty. On that Sunday, we were planning to attend a church located just down the road from our vacation rental apartment. We drove into the parking lot only to be informed that the service was nearing conclusion. The deacon who spoke with us advised us of another church service that he believed we could probably make if we immediately drove down the road about ten more miles, to Haleiwa town.

We set off for Haleiwa, fully expecting to attend the recommended service, but God had other plans in store for us that morning. As we passed by Haleiwa Park on the out-skirts of town, we both noticed a fairly large gathering with tents and grills set up. Then I spotted a sign that said, "We Celebrate Jesus." I said to Mark, "We celebrate Jesus too!" And Mark replied, "Yes, we do," as he quickly navigated the car into the parking lot.

What we discovered that day laid a foundation for a future effort on our own island of Kauai. It also connected the "Once-a-Month Church" Pastor, Ron Valenciana, with Pastors from independent churches who fellowship monthly on Oahu, including Kauai Bible Church. We fully believe that this didn't happen by accident. Again, we see more evidence of God using *all* things, even this cancer treatment trip, for the good of those who love him.

Entry 57
More great news

Subject: **More great news: Val and Mark**
Date: **Sun 06/22/08 10:55 PM**

Aloha everyone!

We just got more great news...on two fronts. First, Val had her bone scan, and it was NORMAL. No evidence of cancer in the structural system! Additionally, we consider it a miracle that sister Susan Willman, M.D., was able to set-up a consultation for a re-evaluation (2nd opinion) of Val's case with an oncologist on Oahu that was highly recommended by a famous cancer specialist in the Bay Area of CA. This will allow confirmation on the chemotherapy that is appro-priate for Val. (Val was originally turned down by the office but Dr. Sue made the phone call to pursue an appointment... and got it on the day Val and Mark would be on Oahu for additional appointments: Truly a miracle!)

Also...the "LIVESTRONG" bracelets are IN!! We just received our order yesterday, so we will be sending them out to those of you who e-mailed us to let us know that you wanted one, or more! If you would like us to send one to you and haven't yet sent us your address and request, please e-mail us, and we will send it out ASAP!

We appreciate all of you standing with us, marching into this battle, and claiming VICTORY!!

Blessings and Love,

* Val and Mark *

P.S. We have attached a note about the bracelets, describing what they are and what they mean to us.

The following is a description of our version of "LIVING **STRONG**." We called it, "LIVE**STRONG** in Jesus!"

The "LIVESTRONG" Bracelets are in!

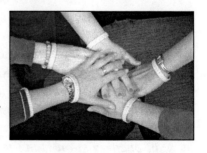

We are excited that we can incorporate these incred-ible representations of VICTORY over cancer into our battle, and we invite you to join us. Our own identification with Lance Armstrong as

*an athlete, "unprecedented-ly" victorious within the field of Professional Cycling, (as well as a courageous cancer survivor with an incredible account of successfully fighting for his life), has lead us to find hope and motivation to "band" together as a team in conquering this notorious foe. Our own twist on the "LIVESTRONG" approach is to, "LIVESTRONG in JESUS!" The Scripture verse we chose for our foundation is Val's favorite; **Philippians 4:13, NKJV,** "I can do all things through Christ who strengthens me." How wonderfully appropriate for this focus on HIS strength for this battle.*

We want to thank our dear friend from Kauai Bible Church, Bunny, who gave us financing to support this effort. God provides for all our needs through His unending supply, and sometimes, that takes the form of the Church family.

We appreciate you ALL. Thank you for "banding together" with us to take a final stand against cancer. We have one request from you, as you wear this bracelet and are reminded to pray, please pray for not only us, but the many, many people who are and will be diagnosed with this disease. The day that our exceptional surgeon gave us the great news that she had successfully removed Val's cancer without any indication of further spread, she disclosed to us that she had the sad task of informing 3 ladies that same week, (one of them a good friend of hers), of very bad news related to their cancers. It gave us a sobering perspective, reminding us that it is only by His great grace and mercy, through all of your prayers that we are on the path to recovery today. We request that you place "#3" on your bracelet somewhere, reminding you to pray for these ladies, and all who precede and follow them.

Thank you, thank you, thank you…so very much. We love and appreciate you all more than we can say. Claiming Victory as we march into this battle with trust and confidence in our Lord Jesus Christ,

Val and Mark

If you are interested in discovering more about the "Lance Armstrong Foundation" go to:

www.livestrong.org

Entry 58
A Visit from the American Cancer Society Representative

I finally decided that I wanted to avail myself of every avenue of support that seemed appropriate. I called the office of the American Cancer Society, (ACS), and they sent Susan Campbell to my home.

Susan is a cancer survivor who volunteers to meet with those diagnosed with the disease. In her visit she was very knowledgeable and gracious. She invited me to discuss anything and everything about her own experience as well as my apprehensions pertaining to treatment.

I was gifted with a very special pillow in the shape of a heart, a sewing project that another cancer survivor completed as her way of demonstrating support for people like me. Then Susan gave me booklets of information pertaining to my situation, and offered to return any time I needed to talk. Finally, she told me about a seminar that the ACS was beginning to offer on Kauai. The seminar was entitled, "Look good: feel better." It was something that I eventually attended and was tremendously blessed by.

Entry 59
CT scan and EKG

This week was particularly busy for me. Life really changes when you receive a cancer diagnosis. It seemed that the health care profession did nothing short of whipping into action on my behalf. I took comfort in this, believing that everything that could be done to help me was being done.

For the CT (Computed Tomography) Scan, I was asked to drink a heavy, goopy solution the night prior, and the morning of my scan. I attempted to specify that this iodine solution should *not* contain sugar, if at all possible, but this effort was in vain. I suffered the consequences the next day with a sugar fatigue that was close to debilitating for my poor body that had not seen any simple sugar in many moons.

At any rate, the scanning went fine. Then I trotted down the hall to wait my turn for an EKG, (Electrocardiogram). The purpose of this test was to determine if my heart was healthy enough to withstand the effects of certain chemicals used in chemotherapy treatment for cancer. It made me suspicious, although my tests came out fine. I have a minor heart condition called, "mitral valve prolapse." It is generally not something to be concerned about, however, under the circumstances, I wondered if I should at least mention the heart palpitations that I was experiencing with increasing frequency. As I would discover later in my journey, there were some chemical treatments that, due to this condition, would probably be best for me to avoid.

Entry 60
Arm rehab-Scans complete

As my arm healed from the surgeries, it became apparent that there was a small problem with my range of motion. The arm felt pretty good, but I really had to strain to raise it above my head. Dr. Emilia gave me a referral to a trusted friend and awesome physical therapist, Dan Schaal. Dan had worked with me on my leg problems in July and August of 2007. He was actually the one who finally figured out that it was a circulatory problem and not a spinal nerve related issue.

I went to Dan and he gave me some exercises designed to improve my arm range of motion. I dutifully performed the exercises but after two days my spinal cord injury had flared up. My neck and back felt the old familiar pain, and I knew that I would not be able to continue this venue for arm restoration. I decided to run an idea past Dan.

My idea was to use baton twirling to rehabilitate my arm. It may sound funny, but I reasoned, "My body *knows* twirling!" Dan agreed that it was worth a shot, and I decided as soon as we returned from our vacation, I would drag those trusty old sticks out and see what happened.

In the meantime, we were presented with the rest of my body scanning and heart test outcomes...all wonderful news! Here is the e-mail we sent after receiving the results:

Subject: Done scanning Val and all is well!
Date: Thu 06/26/08 09:48 PM

Aloha all!

We are VERY happy to report that all the scanning has been completed, and there was no additional sign of cancer through Val's body. Thank you for all your prayers and support! Our next step is to get our re-evaluation and clear direction for chemotherapy that is appropriate for Val. We are leaving tomorrow to fly over to Oahu, where we will see our Naturopathic M.D. as well as an oncologist. Our prayer request is that our doctors be graced with God's wisdom and direction, specifically for Val.

Then we plan on having FUN!! We will be on Oahu for two days staying on the Northshore, and then we fly over to the Island of Lanai. We will be staying there over our 18th anniversary, celebrating and praising the Lord for all he has done in our lives and our marriage. Then for the final two days we will be on Maui. We realize that we are SO blessed being able to travel to all these famous vacation places...right here on our islands. Unbelievable! We hope that each of you from the mainland and our neighboring islands, will someday be able to visit us here on Kauai, and possibly take in another island as well. You ALL have a place to stay whenever you visit us.

We will update you as it becomes clear what direction we will be marching into this battle...Claiming Victory and Praising Jesus!

Love you all!

* Val and Mark *

Entry 61
Dr. Yee is for me!

Within the first few minutes of my initial appointment with Dr. Arnold Yee, I knew that he was our answered prayer. He was God's choice to be my oncologist. Dr. Yee was not only willing to receive, but he actually invited input about our eastern medical approach with Dr. Lam. He eagerly took the bundle of information that I handed him, and immediately began perusing the materials. Rather than dictating a treatment direction founded solely on impersonal statistics from research based on the typical case, he listened carefully to who I was. You cannot imagine the relief I felt as he placed the decision-making process back into our hands.

Dr. Yee had a propensity for complete explanation. For two Ph.D.'s from scientific backgrounds, (Mark's Ph.D. is in agronomy and mine is in psychology), this was quite a bonus. He even printed out a "survival rate chart" to illustrate the typical chances of cancer metastasizing in a variety of different treatment choices. Dr. Yee explained to me that the target survival percentage for most patients is 90%. It appeared that without any individualization whatsoever, I would be starting at the 67% survival position. At this point I became determined to discover a way to gain the additional 23%.

I had always been athletic, exercising almost daily. That added to my survival percentage. Since my diagnosis, I had reduced my simple sugar intake to practically nothing; diet changes add percentage points as well. My non-traditional treatments for hormonal components, (my cancer was determined to be estrogen and progesterone receptor positive, indicating that hormones contributed to the problem), presumably added percentage points. I was also on supplements for decreasing abhorrent cell activity and building immunity, and that should additionally affect the percentages. And then there were Dr. Lam's treatments…a virtual unknown.

In the office that afternoon I determined that I would seek the information that would reveal my true, individualized survival percentage. Then we would see clearly which path of treatment would be appropriate for me.

Dr. Yee was not threatened by this approach. On the contrary, he seemed engaged and eager to learn right along with me. I knew that truly, Dr. Yee was for me!

Entry 62
April: a person of hope

There is a special person I want to introduce you to who represents many that I have met in my journey through cancer. She is actually a nurse for Dr. Yee. Her name is April Goya. April is a tiny lady with respect to physique, but she is a gentle giant of support and hope.

April battled cancer…and won. She went through the dreaded mastectomy surgery, and also chemotherapy. She lost her beautiful black hair, but marched through the process with dignity and strength. As she will tell you, God blessed her with even thicker hair as it grew back in!

April is a beacon of hope within what can be a very dark time in cancer patients' lives. As people enter through the doors of Dr. Yee's office, they are generally seeking ammunition for their battle with cancer. April is a symbol of victory over cancer. Her willingness to discuss any aspect of her personal experiences is a wonderful and unexpected treasure within this medical office context.

She also shares my faith in Jesus. We have spent many moments sharing our stories of how the Lord has wonderfully blessed us. I cherish her friendship and appreciate her willingness to be Jesus' arms to those he sends in to Dr. Yee's office.

Entry 63
E-mail update

Here is the e-mail that we sent upon our return from our trips:

Subject:
Updating you and claiming our Miracle! (Val and Mark)
Date: Sat 07/12/08 09:46 PM

Aloha all!!

We wanted to update you on our recovery progress and plans, as well as share our joy in celebrating our 18th wed-

ding anniversary. As we indicated in our last e-mail, we flew to Oahu and checked in with Dr. Lam, our Naturopathic M.D., who indicated that Val's progress was substantial. Her "Bio-Age" (an indication of her biological functioning, and the body's rebuilding process of her immune system, which attacks the cancer cells), is now normal! This means that her system is at optimal functioning, able to continue working on elimination of any unhealthy cells.

In addition, we met with Dr. Arnold Yee, the oncologist who our sister from California connected us with. Val said, "Dr. Yee is for me!" We both appreciated him so very much. He was able to show us the research and statistics that apply to situations like Val's, and offer us many directions for treatment. He offered to walk through with us, whatever direction we choose. What a freeing and empowering experience! We are grateful for this connection, and his input. He was even open to learning about the naturopathic treatments of Dr. Lam as well as all the supplements that Val has been taking for building her immunity, and attacking the cancer cells via hormone blocking and unhealthy cell destruction. He acknowledged that Val has been improving her statistical probability of successfully beating the cancer through ALL of these different methods of treatment, as well as her determination to affect the cells by NOT providing them with their "preferred" fuel...simple sugars! (Val has been on a very strict "sugar-free" diet since the second day of her diagnosis...this includes eliminating all fruits and processed grains like white rice...hard to do here in Kauai!) It was so good to finally have someone in the medical profession, who was trained in western medical approaches, who would show an interest in learning, and actually connect what we have been doing with an increased success rate! We are so appreciative.

Dr. Yee ordered a blood test for cancer markers, so that we can monitor Val's progress, making sure that there are no indications in her system that the cancer is returning. Our first report verified what we already knew...there are NO indications of cancer in her bloodstream. We praise God and thank you all for the prayers and support that have fostered this miracle of healing! God IS faithful, and by his grace and mercy, Val IS healed.

Our plans for the next two months are to continue with Dr. Lam's treatments. We will be traveling twice in those months to Oahu to check in with both Dr. Lam and Dr. Yee. We will be discussing results of the blood tests and any further exams that Dr. Yee determines are appropriate to monitor Val's progress. After that time, we will make a decision regarding the necessity of further treatment.

Now for the FUN STUFF! We celebrated our 18th anniversary on the small Island of Lanai...known for its resorts and relaxed, laid-back atmosphere. We stayed at Manele Bay Resort, and were absolutely spoiled rotten! What a fabulous place! We were even treated by God to an incredible performance by several pods of "spinner dolphins" right out our back yard in the bay! Val, with her baton twirling trained eye, counted the spins and identified the "five-spin tricks, along with the five spins with an inversion flip!" It was such a blessing. We hiked, swam, snorkeled, Mark went scuba diving, Val went shopping, we were pampered and relaxed tremendously! It was just perfect for us at this time. Most of all, we were thankful for how the Lord restored our marriage. After two and a half years of separation, he brought us both to our knees, and began a powerful reconnection with him as well as with each other. That was 13 years ago, and he has blessed us tremendously by using our experiences to provide encouragement and hope to other couples. What a privilege!

We hope this update finds you and yours well, joy-filled, and being blessed tremendously! We continue claiming victory in this battle, praying for God's mercy and grace for the "three" and all who are affected by cancer. Thanks again for joining with us. We appreciate you all so much.

Love and Blessings,

* Val and Mark *

Entry 64
Lanai anniversary trip (6/29/2008 -7/4/2008)

Part of the reason we decided to indulge ourselves in a resort vacation was that we had to cancel our traditional plans to spend our anniversary in Oregon with my folks. For many years we had spent some time visiting my parents just prior to our anniversary. Then we would get away for a couple of days to be alone together and celebrate our actual anniversary date, which was June 30th. This year was different. We just couldn't leave Hawaii where all my health care professionals were located.

At first it was very disappointing. I was the reason for much of our cancelled plans, and felt guilty because of it. Mark, as usual, took the negative and twisted it into a positive. He said something that we say here in Kauai, "Lucky we live Hawaii!"

There was an element of reality in our decision making process, and that included the fact that cancer is an unpredictable, unknown element. Even with our assuredness via our steadfast faith in the ability for our God to heal, and the awareness that I had received my healing, we still battled the doubts. We reasoned internally that it was possible we would not have many more, if any, anniversaries together. I say internally because it was not spoken aloud. The thought that God just might be calling me home through this process was at the outer edge of my thoughts, and most likely Mark's as well.

We threw finances to the wind and decided to "go for it" in Lanai! This attitude brought to mind the phrase, "live as if you were to die tomorrow...love as if you were to live forever." Cancer helps you do that.

Manele Bay Resort

Mark and I are not "resort people." We found it very difficult to accept the fact that at Manele Bay, there was a staff hired specifically for catering to your every need. I found myself sneaking down the hallway in several futile attempts to get my own ice, only to be busted by a watchful bell-person who would say, "No, no, Mrs. Willman, let *me* get your ice for you!" After my fourth attempt I finally gave up and henceforth called room service to fill my ice bucket.

Mark was more successful at this unauthorized "helping out" than I, discovering his niche in the exercise room. In order to listen to music or hear the audio portion of your private television that was attached to each exercise machine, you had to use a specific type of headphone. After using the headphones, you were supposed to put them into a solution where the staff would meticulously clean each one, and replace it for the next guest. Mark determined that the fitness room staff had plenty to do without having to clean his earphones, so he took his set with him upon finishing his work out. He would then bring his borrowed headphones with him each time, thus helping to eliminate some of what he deemed "unnecessary" service work.

I think we both tried hanging up our once-used towels in such a way as to appear perfectly clean and ready for use. This tactic was for naught as twice *per day* the housekeeping staff came and replaced every single towel in the entire room, whether it had been used or not.

Oh, and the room! Besides boasting a lush "tropical theme in warm golden tones enhanced by rich cherry and rattan furnishings," (taken from the description on the Manele Bay web site), they also had a huge marbled bathroom with a soaking tub and a shower! I realize that I am now sounding like an advertisement for the Resort, but to me, this place is worth touting. (By the way, we did get a "Kama'aina rate" which is a reduced rate for people "of the land": those living in Hawaii.)

Here is the web-site. Check it out for yourself!

http://www.fourseasons.com/manelebay/

Because I had been on my sugar restricted diet, I recognized that eating in this extravagant place could pose a significant challenge. The night we arrived, we went to the main dining room, the Hulopo'e Court. (The name reflects the name of the Ocean Bay that hugs the Resort property.)

When the waiter came to our table we began to describe my limitations, including no white flour, no white rice, no potato, no fruit, no honey, and no sugar of any kind. I then shared with him the reason behind the apparent madness. I told him that I was diagnosed with cancer, and that this was one way we were starving active cancer cells of their preferred fuel. The waiter promptly excused himself and returned moments later with the Maître d', who took out a pen and writing pad and swiftly listed everything we enumerated. He assured us that his chef would make certain that my dinner would not include any of the contaminants. There was confidence conveyed by this man's tone and posture that elicited complete trust from both of us: For very good reason.

During the remainder of our stay, we were treated to astonishing sugar free delicacies, from appetizers and bread, (yes, sugar free bread!), to main courses and salads. Chef even created sugar free desserts to *die for*! (Maybe I better say, to *live* for!) Each evening we were approached by the Maître d' asking us if we planned on dining with them during the next day. We would examine our schedule and decide which meals we could partake of. (Actually, we would look down at our waistlines to check just how much more deliciously rich and extravagant gastronomical delights our bodies could absorb!)

Maybe anyone with dietary restrictions would've been treated with this type of pandering...and maybe not. There is something that should be crystallizing for you as you read about my personal experiences. Cancer extracts compassion from people. It knits their hearts together and induces benevolence. God snatches victory from the jaws of defeat. For me, cancer has been an unfathomable blessing.

Entry 65
Emma

One day during our vacation we decided to visit the sister resort on Lanai, called the "Lodge at Koele." Because most all of the island is owned by David Murdock, via his acquisition of the Castle & Cooke Company, there is a relationship between the two resorts. This allows guests to travel between and use both facilities without additional charges.

The lovely Lodge is seated high up in the mountainous region of the island. Because Lanai is so small, it only takes about a half hour on a shuttle bus to travel between the two properties. We walked the beautiful gardens, taking pictures of each other, and then found a nice little golf clubhouse restaurant to have lunch.

We were enjoying the view from the terrace overlooking the fabulous golf course when my cell phone rang. It was our friend and conscientious house cleaning helper, Opuulani. She had dropped by our house to check on our cat, Pumpkin. Her message in a nutshell was that Pumpkin had a very bad case of diarrhea. I immediately called our neighbor who was Pumpkin sitting, and relayed the message. I had visions of poor Pumpkin, lonely and sick. (Yes, I am a cat person.)

A few minutes later, Emma called back. She assured me that she would handle any problem that Pumpkin was having, and actually ordered me not to worry. Emma is a nurse. She has a heart of pure gold and a gift of compassionate giving that is second to none. I knew Pumpkin's needs would be met, and they were.

The real reason I am introducing you to Emma is not to expose you to our feline's elimination difficulties. I actually want to tell you about something Emma did after we returned from Lanai.

When Emma heard about my cancer diagnosis, she determined that she would make me a Haku Lei, (a Hawaiian head ornament). She desired to do something, and this gesture she knew would touch me. The major road block to making the lei was that she did not know how. One day Emma was talking to a lady who was hospitalized for cancer and she discovered that this woman was willing to teach her how to make a Haku Lei. Emma told me that she put off learning for a while, because her time consuming job demanded attention. Then one day Emma went into the woman's room only to discover that the woman had passed away from the cancer. The experience so shocked Emma that she urgently vowed to learn how to make the lei...before it was too late to give it to me.

When we returned from Lanai, not only was Pumpkin doing very well, but Emma had made a beautiful Haku Lei from lovely miniature roses that she harvested from her own back yard. It was precious and so was her desire to communicate how very much she cared. People do these things when they discover you have cancer. There is an urgent imploring that is triggered by this notorious diagnosis. In a way, it draws the best out of people.

We swam, snorkeled, hiked, shopped, (well... I shopped), exercised, ate and enjoyed our anniversary tremendously. God really spoiled us rotten during our time on Lanai. It was actually a horrible let-down as we left the island and traveled to Maui. There we stayed in a regular hotel room where we actually had to bring in our own luggage!

Now as I pull up the Manele Bay web site and gaze at the picture taken from the main lobby of the resort, looking out onto the bay, I feel the peace and joy of our wonderful, extravagant anniversary trip. And to think that I could've missed out on it, had I not been diagnosed with cancer! Darlene calls it "lemonade." She says, "Lemon, lemon, lemonade! Squeeze those lemons that life hands you, and make more lemonade!" This Lanai lemonade was a very sweet variety that wasn't polluted with forbidden sugars!

Entry 66
Researching treatments

When we returned from our vacation I dove into the literature looking for those elusive, survival percentage points and appropriate directions for treatment. I spent hours and hours combing through articles from government websites and educational institutions. I scoured reports from non-traditional places such as natural product information outlets and eastern health practice resources. I accumulated stacks of information and copious lists of websites.

At the same time my dad was doing something similar with the resources he was familiar with. One day he sent the culmination of his efforts to me in the mail. There were just two pages copied. They looked like they could've come from the "National Enquirer Magazine." But, in those two pages, my intellectually gifted father had identified two prominent directions for cancer treatment. One was vaccination and one was tumor testing. Leave it to my dad to boil things down to the most valuable essence!

I pursued these leads, discovering related research projects being conducted at major universities under government grants. I could hardly wait to show the information to Dr. Yee at our next appointment!

Entry 67
Using baton twirling for rehabilitation

The Hanapepe tennis courts, located directly across the street from the Pacific Ocean, were vacant. I parked my little sport model Toyota Celica with its trunk toward the court. That way the music from my car's CD player would transmit volume via the slight trade wind into my ears. Music always gives me an extra "oomph" of motivation, and this day, I would need it.

There was an uncharacteristic hesitancy in my movements as I slowly began to spin my baton. I carefully avoided twirling patterns that would require my injured arm to stretch in any direction. As I gained more and more confidence, I expanded to include greater arm extension. I kept reminding myself to take it slowly, not something that came naturally for this five-time Grand National Champion twirler. Each time I felt a twinge of pulling on the underside of my arm, I said to myself, "not that twirling move…not yet."

After a while, I was dancing and twirling to my contemporary Christian CD, with absolute joy and ecstasy! I could hardly believe what I was capable of executing only one month after my lymph node surgery and mastectomy! "Thank you, Lord," was the phrase that ruminated in my being.

7/2009

As I practiced twirling over the ensuing weeks, it became obvious to me that God was granting me a desire of my heart. He says that he will:

(*Psalm 37:4* "Take delight in the LORD, and he will give you the desires of your heart.").

I have always described this scripture as having two implications. The first rests on God's ability to implant desires into my heart, thus "giving me" the craving I feel inside. Additionally, I don't believe that God would instill a desire without also providing an opportunity to fulfill that desire. In this case my desire was to twirl for him, worshiping him using my beloved batons in such a way that would give him pleasure, and that I could reciprocally feel his pleasure.

Do you remember a movie called, "Chariots of Fire?" It was based on a true story about Eric Liddell, a Scottish track and field athlete who won gold and bronze medals at the 1924 Olympics. Eric was known for his integrity and Christian faith. During the film there was a scene depicting a disagreement between Eric and his sister. She questioned Eric's motivation to run, arguing that his life direction should be serving as a missionary in China, like their parents. Eric answered that he had every intention of becoming a missionary, but first, he would run. He explained it by telling her, "When I run, I feel God's pleasure."

When I twirl, I feel God's pleasure.

Entry 68
Ukulele classes

Just prior to my diagnosis Mark and I had signed up for free Ukulele classes from a precious Christian woman who attended Lihue Missionary Church. Diane Horita offered the free classes to anyone, and we discovered it when our Associate Pastor and gifted Music Director, David Leong, sent our church e-mail list the announcement. Diane considered it her ministry, using the ukulele venue to teach Christian, Hawaiian and Christmas songs to her groups.

Mark and I borrowed ukuleles and attended classes once per week. We were just beginning to become better acquainted with fellow participants when I received the breast cancer diagnosis. Our reluctance to share our plight with the class was singly related to our lack of familiarity with them. We decided that we needed to disclose, because we did not know how the medical treatment would affect our ability to participate in the group.

Here is yet another example of how God works all things for our good. The small group of ukulele students, along with our lovely teacher, Diane, fell silent as we shared my news. After a few moments of silence, Diane said, "I just feel like we need to gather around Val and pray for her." They all circled around me, laying their hands on me, and praying for everything from peace and comfort to healing. It was such a blessing.

Throughout the eight weeks of ukulele classes, the group supported and prayed for me. Just this week I discovered an e-mail that Diane sent to me. It is very precious as you will discover:

Subject: How are you doing?
Date: Wed 07/09/08 08:50 PM

Hi Val and Mark,

Thank you for your up-date. I'm so glad you were able to travel and enjoy yourselves immensely. I'm glad you took your uku-lele on your trip. I do that too and have made friends just by the music. It also helps to pass the time when there is a delay.

Praise the Lord for the good report so far, and we continue to ask that the Lord strengthen and continue to heal you completely. I hope you are eating and putting on weight too. I should have taught you a Japanese song. Perhaps in the future, Lord willing. There's an easy one, "If You're Happy and You know It, Clap Your Hands".

Praising the Lord is so important when trouble comes our way. Just keep praising the Lord. There was a young lady in ICU once who had had a stroke down at the beach. She was paralyzed on the right side of her body. She had a 5 year old son.

Whenever our hospital ministry went to sing and pray over her, she would lift her left arm heavenward in praise. She could not talk. She did that every time. About a year later, while I was shopping at "Big Save" in Lihue, someone tapped me on the shoulder. It was this young lady. She was walking, talking, and praising the Lord!!!

Please include me in your prayer communication.

Praising the Lord for your healing,

Diane

Diane's encouragement gave my faith a booster shot. When you hear about miracles like the one she described in her e-mail, don't you just gotta believe?!

Entry 69
Nosode treatments

During the month of July Mark dutifully injected me with the chemical nosode treatments from Dr. Lam. For each weekly shot Mark carefully combined the liquids of 14 different vials. Consistent with his character, Mark developed an organized method to accomplish this task. I am uncertain how many loving husbands would have the stomach for jabbing their wife in the leg and then slowly administering a chemical solution. I am grateful for Mark's willingness. I also treasure Mark's family upbringing that associated him with doctors, hospitals and needles, (through his surgeon father), something that God used to prepare him for this season in our lives.

I learned to drink "beaucoup" amounts of water prior to and within 12 hours after each shot. This helped me avoid most of the distasteful side effects. For me the hardest part of this was to relinquish my treasured coffee drinks. I was told by Dr. Lam that it was best to avoid anything that had a strong aroma, especially coffee. In my quest for health and anti-cancer dieting, I had identified that I really enjoyed cold coffee, but during the day before and after my shots, I had to surrender that too.

Of course, I had to test this to be sure that the rules of Dr. Lam truly applied to *me*. One Saturday just after Mark injected me, I decided to allow myself one of my delicious cold coffee mochas, with sugar free chocolate syrup and sweetener. I rationalized that cold coffee really doesn't have a robust smell. Surely it wouldn't affect me the same way that hot coffee would!

Shortly after I downed my treat Mark and I decided to go grocery shopping. On the way to the store, I didn't notice anything different. I was doing just fine, thank you very much! I said, to myself, "Dr. Lam is just being overly cautious with this coffee restriction." We exited our car and walked to where the carts were located. One of our friends was putting away her cart so we stopped to say "Hi." As we did, I thought to myself, "Man! This gal needs some discretion regarding the amount of perfume she uses." After a couple of minutes, I thought I was going to get asphyxiated from the intensity of that fragrance. When we parted from her company I made a smart remark about her perfume, but Mark said he didn't notice anything. I said, "How could you *help* but notice!"

Then we entered the store. At each aisle I noticed someone with such pungent odor that it was actually caustic. I began breathing as shallow as possible, hoping to compensate for everyone else's rude disregard for basic hygiene. When we stepped out the front door into the Kauai sunshine, I thought I was going to go blind! Then my head began to pound and my stomach queezed. Mark and I sat in the car as I gulped as much water as I could, hoping to drown and flush out the effects of my coffee indiscretion.

I learned the hard way that Dr. Lam knew what he was talking about, and that I needed to refrain from having my beloved coffee drinks anywhere near the time of my injections.

Rats! Sometimes obedience can be a real *bummer*!

As we moved closer to our next visit to Dr's Lam and Yee on Oahu, we were blessed with some help on Kauai. From the Kauai Medical Clinic where my heroes, Dr's Penner and Williamson and company are, came an oncologist willing to coordinate our treatment alongside Dr. Yee. Dr. Eileen Denny, a woman who traveled from Oahu once per week to help with the Kauaian oncological needs, generously agreed to help us. She had previously worked with Dr. Yee, and thought a lot of him, so it was a natural, God-ordained connection for us.

Mark and I met with Dr. Denny and described our needs for blood tests and other potential requirements of Dr. Yee's, and she facilitated the process. There is a really funny story I have about the caring and interconnectedness of the Kauai Medical Clinic staff. I will tell you about it next.

Entry 70
Go To The Nearest Emergency Medical Clinic...

This particular morning I had my blood drawn at Kauai Medical Clinic. Each time prior to visiting my doctors on Oahu, Dr. Denny would arrange for me to be vampired, for the purpose of running relevant tests such as cancer markers and immune system indicators. That way when I checked in with my doctors on Oahu there would be objective evidence of my health.

On the island of Kauai, due to the fact that we have a limited amount of resources in the middle of the Pacific Ocean, it is always a crap shoot to get that elusive first place in line for blood drawing. I discovered that if I walked over to the Clinic at 8 a.m. when they open for blood drawing, I might be the first, or I might be the unfortunate one that is too late for the drawing that day. (They draw blood from 8 to 9 a.m., on Monday through Thursday.) I learned to go over early and wait outside the doors to ensure my place in line. It makes me feel kind of rotten as I get first draw while 90 year old "Nanna" who can barely walk up the steps to the clinic, has to wait until her number is called. Such is part of our limited resource island lifestyle.

After my turn that day in the laboratory I scooted home to get ready and make the drive into Lihue for my weekly shopping excursion. I turned on my cell phone, a new one that I happened to be trying out, but it never responded. "That's it!" I exclaimed. "I'm taking the dumb thing back." So off I went to the phone company, anticipating an exchange of phones. It was so busy in the office that I decided to do my shopping first.

It was after noon by the time I returned to the phone company's office. By that time, I had gathered via the "coconut wireless," (an island means of communication and rumor dissemination), that the phone company's service had gone down. I entered the office and was dealing with a representative, when the phone service was reestablished. My phone immediately indicated that I had a message, and I accessed it, turning it on to speaker phone so that I could hear above the noise of multiple customer transactions. Within seconds I heard my dear husband's voice loudly announcing that I should *"Go to the nearest emergency medical clinic!"* He stated that Kauai Medical Clinic had been trying to reach me without luck, so they left a distress message with him. Mark indicated that it was related to my blood test earlier that morning.

By this time I had switched off the loudspeaker function on my phone, but it was too late. The entire office began backing away from me as if they had just discovered I had the swine flu! As I listened to the message again, I determined that there must've been something on the needle that was used to poke me, and I was probably exposed to a contaminant. They wanted me to go to the emergency room upon manifestation of symptoms such as fatigue, (suddenly I was feeling quite tired), fever, (I did begin to sweat profusely), or other such maladies.

As I left the phone company's office I attempted to call Kauai Medical Clinic, but my phone service went out just as I was put on hold to talk to the nurse. I figured that I would just go to the clinic and get the scoop in person.

It was a "lovely" 30 minute ride down the only road that connects Lihue with the west side of the island. I began using my psychological tools for relaxation and stress reduction...oh, *OK*! It was actually for panic minimization! And, of course, I prayed.

When I arrived at the clinic, they got the nurse from in the back room, and ushered me in to the laboratory. The nurse proceeded to ask me several questions regarding the type of cancer treatment I was undergoing. She finally asked me if I was exposed to a virus lately, and I answered that it was possible. To make a long story short, the blood tests were "expedited" by Dr. Denny, as she does for all her cancer patients, and my results revealed a depleted white blood cell count. This indicated a potential infection, something that for people undergoing traditional chemotherapy, can be life threatening. For me, it was simply enlightening, and all out relieving! Yes, I probably did have a cold virus. In fact, my throat was beginning to get sore just thinking about it. But my life was not in danger!

I expelled a huge amount of hot air that had been trapped inside me as I was holding my breath and bracing for potentially horrifying news. I felt much better. Upon review of this whole ordeal, I recognized what an incredible medical support team I had. Oh my...the joys of the cancer diagnoses! But what extraordinary lengths these medical professionals went to on my behalf, to be sure I was safe. These are the unfathomable, unpredictable blessings associated with the diagnosis, and the journey through cancer.

Entry 71
More survival percentage points!

An e-mail was sent to us from Mark's sister, Sarah Cuneo. I rejoiced as I read it. The article she sent us described a study called the CONCORD study. The research population, gathered from 31 countries, included over two million cancer patients, ages 15-99. Professor Michael Coleman, MD, from the London School of Hygiene and Tropical Medicine, was the lead author.

Professor Coleman identified Hawaii as having the best cancer survival rate in the U.S. for breast and colon cancer. All-Right!! I can knock off a few more percentage points from the magic number "23"that I am on the hunt for! It makes sense to me, having lived in the south-eastern part of Washington, central Washington, central Indiana and north-west Indiana, that a climate that maximizes your exposure to the sun, provides an atmosphere where health abounds. Scientists keep coming out with more evidence that vitamin D, something we get naturally via exposure to the sunlight, enhances immunity.

In addition, the pace of life here on Kauai may add to the health picture. There are common phrases voiced by local residents here, such as, "Slow down, this is Kauai," "Ain't no big thing," and "Hang loose," that highlight a popular relaxed attitude. If you can associate primarily with people who apply these principles to their lives, then the stress of living can be significantly less.

Entry 72
Doctor checkups in Oahu

Armed with an overabundance of information from my research, Mark and I departed to Oahu for checkups at Dr. Lam's and Dr. Yee's offices. At Dr. Lam's our major concern involved the trip we were about to take to Puerto Rico. Mark's work was sending him for business meetings, and I was planning to accompany him. The only draw-back was our injection regimen. I was scheduled to receive my monthly dosage during the two weeks we would be traveling. Dr. Lam had previously warned us against trying to take the nosodes on an airplane. He recounted examples of patients getting their precious chemicals confiscated, necessitating a re-order from Germany with accompanying four to six weeks delay in treatment. Fortunately, Dr. Lam assured us that if we waited to proceed with my injections until we returned from our trip, it would suffice. Additionally, he found it necessary to give me a "booster injection" on the spot, ruining my plans to treat myself with a Vietnamese coffee after the appointment.

Later that afternoon, we walked into Dr. Yee's office. I promptly handed him the carefully organized information I had collected, and we were off and running. He listened and simultaneously skimmed the material as I attempted to explain the key components. Once I had illustrated where I had "gained" many of the crucial survival percentage points, I began making my case for a brand new direction in cancer treatment.

I referred to the "Oncotype DX" tumor test, and Dr. Yee quickly stated, "That has not been used in a case like yours." I was ready for that response, as I presented in rapid succession, all the reasons that I believed it would be appropriate for me. He paused...Dr. Yee rarely is rendered speechless, but this was a time for intellectual contemplation and reasoning. My life was on the line, and I knew it.

After what seemed like ages, Dr. Yee slowly stated, "Yes, yes I believe you are right." "This will help us determine whether or not you really need chemotherapy." I began to internally celebrate. He was buying into the idea. Then he added, "I know you, Val." "If this test indicates that you need chemotherapy, you will be the first in line for the treatments." I thought to myself, "first in line?" But knowing myself as I did, he was probably correct. If I really needed to go through traditional chemotherapy, then by all means, bring it on!

Dr. Yee thought it all the way through, recognizing the need to make a case to convince my insurance company that they should pay for this very expensive tumor test. I am still amazed at his insight and willingness to go the extra mile for his patients. As we left that day, we knew God had placed this direction in our path, and we were on it!

Entry 73
Puerto Rico trip: 8/1/08-8/9/08

The trip to Puerto Rico was very relaxing for me. So relaxing that even though I had planned to write in my journal, I never found the energy to do it.

Most of the time I was on my own, as Mark's time was consumed with business engagements. I made full use of the opportunity to explore the country by taking taxi rides into the town of Ponce. I knew just enough Spanish from high school and college, to prompt one of three reactions from the local Puerto Ricans:

1. scowling
2. laughter
3. bewilderment

All reactions were in response to my misuse of the language, and my insistence that I knew what I was talking about. I was grateful that nobody seemed too offended and happy that most people were more than willing to help me navigate whatever mess that I got myself into.

I didn't think about my cancer diagnosis much. I guess it was a respite from my world of health testing and cancer matters. When I was on the Alaskan cruise with my girl-friends two years ago, I adopted a perspective that helped me glean the most out of the experience. I attempted to "live a lifetime" during those days we shared on the cruise ship. I was able to absorb a plethora of memories from that trip by focusing one moment at a time, squeezing every drop of sweetness from each and every experience. I also "lived a lifetime" during our Puerto Rico vacation.

This perspective has become a way of life for me. It is clearly related to a recognition forced by the cancer diagnosis. I gained immediate insight into my own mortality via an obvious but shocking revelation that any moment could potentially be my last opportunity to live this life.

Here is the e-mail that I sent out upon return from our three week trip to Puerto Rico (8/1-8/9/08) and Oregon (8/10-8/18/08).

Subject: Update from Val and Mark
Date: Sat 08/23/08 07:18 PM

Aloha Everyone!

We just returned from a fairly long trip that by God's Grace, we were able to take at this time! Mark's work, Pioneer Hi-Bred (seed), sent him to Puerto Rico for intense meetings with the other Pioneer employees he works in partnership with from around the world. Val went along to play and use her pathetic knowledge of Spanish! It was a good trip, and after that week, we visited Val's parents on the Oregon Coast, in Bandon. That was very busy, as mom and dad had MUCH planned! We had fun, and it was good to see them and let them see how Val is doing too.

Val is doing great! She feels better than she has in many years, and we are confident that there has been a miraculous healing via all your supportive love and prayers. We have received two blood tests that show NO indications of any residual cancerous cell activity. During Val's last visit with Dr. Lam, our naturopathic M.D., he also picked up NO more cancerous cell activity. He even told Val that now that the cancer is gone, she could have some sugar...just not to over-

do it. Val feels convicted that she needs to stay mostly on a sugar-free diet for now, limiting most all sources of simple sugars. (It is nice not to be worrying about the amount of sugar in mayonnaise or salsa though!)

During Val's visit with Dr. Yee, she and the doctor determined that there are a couple of additional tests that may help determine if what Val has been doing for estrogen, (a component identified in the original cancer), has been working. Also, Dr. Yee believes as we do, that there is a test for the tumor itself that can identify whether this tumor is more likely to spread, or less likely to spread. He said he would attempt coordinating efforts to perform this exam. Val will be visiting all her doctors in Oahu next Friday, August 29th.

Our prayer request at this time is for revelation of the miracle healing that has already taken place. We are praying that all her doctors will recognize that God has healed Val, and be in alignment with what we already know is true!

Something else we want to share with you. When we were taking our seats on the airplane from Puerto Rico to Oregon, Val realized that she had forgotten her "pillow" on the car ride to the airport. Those of you who know about Val's accident about three and a half years ago (when her neck lost stability for an instant - much like a whiplash event - while twirling batons for the "Great Kaua'i Weigh-out" at the local mall) know that since that time, Val has carried this pillow with her wherever she goes. There has not been a time when she traveled anywhere, or sat anytime, without it or at least some back support. The doctors who worked with Val (we lost count at 11), told her this would be something she would have to adjust to for the rest of her life. It seems that pillow became the "savior" for Val in her neck and back trauma, as it helped control the pain. We knew that someday, it would be inevitable, that the poor old thing would either be lost or just fall apart...what we did not know, is how dramatically it would affect Val.

As the realization of what was happening set in, Val began to lose it! She had visions of the past three and a half years spinning in her head. She felt the loss of this "savior" that she had relied on for comfort and support. Then the recognition that airline travel had been the most difficult of any sitting over the years, and that now, on this international flight, she would be left without it. Also, she thought of how her parents loved to take her and Mark on long car rides over the "roller coaster" like roads of the Oregon coast. Those swirvey, windey roads always took a toll on her neck and back, but the pillow was a great help. As the tears rolled off Val's face, Mark dove for his phone, and called the limo company, arranging for the pillow to be sent back to Kauai... but Val knew, the rest of the trip would be without it.

Then something that God had been working on with Val came into her mind..."Bidden or unbidden, God is present." (We originally saw this printed in Latin on a sign that was hanging over Dr. Dan Dye's office in Richland, WA. Val had worked with Dan during the time we spent in Richland before coming to Kauai.) She began to pray, saying, "it's now just you, God. I have no options here, and I bid you come forth and help me now."

Very interesting how God works. Val would have NEVER given up that pillow willingly. Had this never happened, she would not have experienced the healing that God had for her...of her neck and back pain. There was no strange feeling, no warm sensation as we have heard of, but what transpired demonstrated that the promise given at the begin-

ning of this spinal cord injury, was fulfilled. The promise was, "No weapon formed against you will prosper." (Sound familiar?!) Anyway, Val has not experienced the pain in her neck and back as she had for the past three and a half years. She has not used any substitute "saviors" and has been able to lean back and relax in chairs, where this was proclaimed by her doctors to NOT BE POSSIBLE!! We know that "With God, all things are possible." It seems Val needed to remember who her TRUE savior was, and rely on him and him alone. We are claiming this as another miracle healing in Val's life, only by God's grace and mercy.

We hope that all of you are doing great! We continue praying that you receive DOUBLE PORTIONS of the Blessings that you are providing in our lives. As they say here in Kauai, "Mahalo Nui Loa...thank- you very much!"

We love you all,

* Val and Mark *

Entry 74
Port flushing

As soon as we returned to Kauai, I returned to my cancer reality. There was a tiny matter of the "port" my breast surgeon had placed into my body in anticipation of chemotherapy. It was a devise designed to allow easy access for chemical transfusion. The devise required a monthly flushing to ensure free-flowing usability. This was the second trip that I had made to the Wilcox Hospital infusion room.

During the first flushing I made the mistake of sharing my story in detail, including the belief that I had been healed. Well-meaning nurses found it necessary to educate me on what they believed was the absolutely essential component for any cancer treatment regimen, chemotherapy. As I shared my "Dr. Lam treatments" and my research pertaining to tumor testing, I was quite clearly presented the all too familiar message, "If you do what they say to do, you will surely die." It's funny how God can change things, virtually overnight.

This monthly visit was different. The day prior to my port flush appointment the hospital had offered training to their staff, introducing the brand new tumor test procedure. Instead of fierce opposition to my treatment direction, I was validated and encouraged. What a difference! I believe that somehow, God allowed these contrasting port flush experiences as a metaphorical illustration of how dramatically and rapidly he can change things. It served as confirmation of God's hand in what was yet to unfold...

Entry 75
Oncotype results

This day is one I will always remember. I flew to Oahu to see each of my three medical doctors; Dr. Wong, Dr. Yee and Dr. Lam. The day is recorded in my little appointment book as, "Dr.'s Day in Oahu." I scheduled my one year checkup for my leg angioplasty surgery with Dr. Wong that morning, and planned to check in with Dr. Yee in the afternoon. The following day I would see Dr. Lam. Mark had decided to stay in Kauai this time, expecting status quo.

My meeting with Dr. Wong went smoothly. My leg was progressively healing, therefore, most of our conversation centered on my cancer journey. James Wong was on our "Victory Over cancer" e-mail list, fully appraised of our experiences. Consequent of all we had walked through via today's e-mail universe, my cancer diagnosis provided an opportunity for a more intimate connection. It's amazing how God uses the cancer experience to generate infinitely more from every relationship. Those who experience the diagnosis will have the opportunity to fully appreciate this surprising blessing.

My appointment with Dr. Yee was scheduled for 4:30pm. As I entered the office, I was whisked into the hallway where a nurse took my vitals. Then she informed me that my Oncotype DX Breast Cancer Assay score was in. My initial reaction was, "In what?" I had no idea that the tumor testing could happen so quickly. After all, Dr. Yee would have to first get in touch with my breast surgeon, then the hospital, then he would need to contact the laboratory where my original tumor was located, then have the tumor tested at a different laboratory, alongside dealing with my insurance company, and to be completely transparent, these things just take time, especially in Hawaii! I was dumbfounded. This nurse told me that she did not know how to read the test score, so I would have to wait for the Doctor.

It had not even occurred to me that this might be happening today. I had no opportunity to prepare myself by fretting and obsessing over the past month while all these events were taking place on my behalf. I did attempt to make up for this oversight on my part by creating a sharp spike in my adrenal production, increasing my heart rate and blood pressure to an "appropriate peak of anticipation anxiety." By the time Dr. Yee called me into his office, I could barely move.

Dr. Yee said, "Your test results indicate a score of 4." I said, "For...what?" He said, "This indicates that you do not need chemotherapy." I felt a rush of elation ripping through my being. I stated, "So what you are telling me is that God has performed a miraculous healing in me, and I do not need chemotherapy?" Dr. Yee replied, "Yes, God has performed a miracle in you and you do not need chemotherapy." All I remember after receiving that news was "high- fiveing" the Doctor, and then hugging anyone who was in the hallway and behind the reception desk. They were also giving each other "high fives" because as I learned shortly thereafter, they were all involved in making this test happen. There were receptionists who made calls to Kauai, coordinating efforts to obtain samples of the tumor. There were also medical personnel who actually picked up the sample at one laboratory, and delivered it to another. It was an office project, and an office victory.

It was finished. God had answered our most difficult prayer...to get all my doctors into agreement. From eastern medical practitioners to western medical practitioners, they were all in agreement. God *had* performed a miraculous healing in me, and I did not need chemotherapy!

Entry 76
Do you believe in miracles? Yes!

Here is the e-mail that Mark and I sent out making the announcement:

Subject:
Do you believe in miracles??? YES!! (Val and Mark)
Date: Tue 09/02/08 09:52 PM

Dear Everyone:

We are ecstatic and overwhelmed as the Lord has answered ALL of our prayers. Val will not be requiring chemotherapy. All of our doctors, from east, non-traditional approaches, to west, traditional perspectives, agree; there has been a miraculous healing and God has healed Val of the cancer. As you are all very aware, this is exactly what we asked that you pray for, and what we requested from our Lord.

Val traveled to Oahu to see her doctors this weekend. The last time she saw her oncologist, Dr. Yee, it was agreed that there was a test that would help identify the potential for metastasis of the cancer. The test is called, the Oncotype-DX, an assay for breast cancer. Dr. Yee agreed that this test would be appropriate for Val's particular case, and he stated that he would do all he could to see that the insurance would cover it. (The test involves testing material from the tumor, and identification of gene sequences within the DNA.) We did not expect this test to be performed by the time Val went back this weekend...we were happily wrong!

Dr. Yee had arranged with his staff to coordinate the testing, and by the time Val arrived, the results were in. To make a long story short, Dr. Yee informed Val, with a huge smile on his face, that her score was 4...out of 100. When Val asked what that meant, he announced that it meant she did not need chemotherapy. Val said, "So what you are saying is that we are now all in agreement that God has performed a miracle healing and I do not need chemotherapy." Dr. Yee said, "Yes, God has performed a miracle, and you do not need chemotherapy." It seemed that the entire office was involved in obtaining the sample from Kauai, coordinating the test, and running around Oahu transferring materials and finally receiving the results. There were hugs all around, high 5's and praising God for his mercy and grace.

When Val left the office, she spent a few moments reflecting on the many components that had to come together for this miracle to come full circle. From the day that we left the office of an oncologist in Kauai who refused to learn about Val's case as an individual; recommending hard core chemotherapy, and possibly additional radiation when the chemo was completed...to much concerted effort at prayer and direction, to calls via sister (and Dr.) Susan Willman, who identified an oncologist on Oahu who turned out to be an answer to MUCH prayer...to an incredible amount of research on new approaches to cancer treatment by Val and her dad, Don Ludwick...to Dr. Yee's open minded willingness to learn and walk alongside us to identify the right treatment for Val...to the identification of the Oncotype-DX, and it's brand new, appropriate application to Val's particular case...to Dr. Yee's office and their efforts to obtain permission and then coordinate the testing...WOW!!! We've come a LONG way, baby!

We believe that the result of this event is much more of a miracle than the healing itself. Our belief is that Val was healed during the time between her two surgeries. It was during that time when we all banded together and fully engaged in a FIGHT against this cancer. With our Church, Kauai Bible Church, fasting and praying for three days prior to the second surgery, (as well as Val's mom and dad, and a few other folks who heard about this effort), in addition to all your prayers and support, the cancer really did not stand a chance. It was the ALIGNMENT of all the doctors involved...from east to west...all in agreement, and recognition that there WAS a miraculous healing for Val, that we have prayed for since then; THAT was such an incredible miracle! If only you all could have been in the offices and heard the doctors, nurses, technicians and more, from both sides, pointing at each other saying, "If you do what THEY say, you will die!" How much further away can anyone get from alignment?! We know our God, and we know that he can do ANYTHING.

What now? We finish up the shots from Dr. Lam, (three more), and continue with the supplements Val has been on to block unhealthy estrogen and improve immune system functioning as well as reduce abhorrent cell activity, all under the direction and advise of Dr. Yee. Val's next checkup will be in about three months. It is so nice to not have uncertainty hanging over us. We are so thankful.

Again, you must all take a bow for being willing to fight this battle alongside us. The role you have played in the Victory is one we will forever be grateful to you for. We love you all and look forward to your visits, e-mails, phone calls or any way you can stay in contact. Our prayers for you include that the Lord will pour out DOUBLE portions of Blessings to you for all the Blessings you have provided to us.

You cannot know how much we appreciate you all. We will ask God to confirm it in your hearts.

Aloha Blessings and Love,

* Val and Mark *

Entry 77
Embodiment of the miracle

We basked in the glow of God's miracle over the next few months. Every three months since that time we have traveled to Oahu to check in with my doctors, and every time we have been given confirmation of the healing. My twirling rehabilitation project has been transformed into a ministry over the past year. I am so very grateful that God allows me to use this gift to praise and glorify him, and to encourage others.

My first opportunity to embody the miracles of healing I have been blessed with, through my twirling, came during my birthday weekend, October, 2008. "Pastor Appreciation Day" was celebrated at Kauai Bible Church. I wanted to contribute something special to the program to honor our pastors as well as our church family that had battled cancer so valiantly. I saw it as a chance for us all to claim the victory together. I also wanted to thank the lovely women in my women's Bible study group. Nancy Stack, (our amazing Bible study leader), included my dance and twirl routine in her program that same week.

I performed to the song, "Thank you for giving to the Lord," by Ray Boltz. Here is a link to the video of my performance at Kauai Bible Church, taken by a wonderful church sister, Suzan Glantz:

http://www.youtube.com/watch?v=kpRc09FWuCY

The words were perfect to convey Mark's and my desired message, "Thank you for giving to the Lord. I am a life that was changed. Thank you for giving to the Lord, I am so glad you gave."

God's restoration of my body made this performance possible. The performance demonstrated God's healing miracles in a powerful manner. It was a God ordained way to tell everyone thank you for the role they played in claiming the victory over cancer. Thanks to Suzan's taping of the performance, I believe it still is.

Entry 78
9/11/2009

I just realized what today's date is. I am sure that I am not the only one who recalls exactly where I was and what I was doing when I heard about the attack on the Twin Towers in New York City.

I was getting ready to teach my psychology laboratory class at Valparaiso University. One of my colleagues darted out into the hallway and notified us of the disaster and impending dangers that were continuing to loom above the skies of the eastern United States. What a horrifying time in our history that day was. The attack seemingly unraveled our sense of security and our notions of reality in our little worlds, cutting to the core of our identity as Americans.

Dan Wolgemuth, President of Youth for Christ/USA, in his Friday message that just happened to fall on this year's infamous date, addressed a moment such as this from a very unique perspective.

Dan Wolgemuth: President Youth for Christ/USA: September 11, 2009

Most of us have been a witness to a gifted athlete savoring a significant accomplishment with a protracted pause. A baseball player whose position remains fixed at home plate after he clobbers a significant home run. A young tennis player who stands on the baseline after hitting the match-winning top spin passing shot. The wide receiver who makes a stellar catch in the end zone and stands for a moment to relish the accomplishment.

Significant moments invite us to linger; to listen to the crowd; to cherish the spotlight.

Lingering squeezes every last drop out of the experience. It refuses to move on, without first staying put... for the moment. Yes, every wonderful, celebratory, victorious, heroic milestone demands a linger.

But what if the intent of God is for us to do the same lingering when the crowd is silent; when the score isn't in our favor; when somebody else is the hero; when we have more pain than joy; more questions than answers? Is it possible that one of the most significant marks of a follower of Christ is that they have learned not to race through the problems... but to linger there as well... in the chaos, in the suffering, in the battle... because it is there, perhaps especially there, that God meets us.

Is it possible to reject the notion that, "When the going gets tough, the tough get going!" What if we linger when the going gets tough? Not paralyzed, but reflective. Not frozen, but thoughtful. Not hopeless, but expectant. Not defeated, but humble.

Standing, waiting, extracting... the nectar that resides in the deepest part of pain and uncertainty; because we lingered. In the moment. With the moment.

"Come to me..." – this precious invitation of Jesus is designed for those with courage enough to linger... not on the podium of a champion, but on the battlefield of the warrior.

Linger... God is there.

(Reprinted with permission)

Could it be that even in the depths of darkness that *is* the cancer diagnosis, there is something to be gained? If you have continued reading this journal, then you already know what I think.

My favorite part of this article is where Dan describes the reason we might consider "lingering" in an experience such as cancer:

"Is it possible that one of the most significant marks of a follower of Christ is that they have learned not to race through the problems... but to linger there as well... in the chaos, in the suffering, in the battle... because it is there <u>perhaps especially there</u>, that God meets us."

From one who has been *"there,"* let me share the truth with you. God met me, over and over again. He is no respecter of person, and he will do for you what he did for me.

I love how Dan finishes his article with the invitation of Jesus, to linger, with courage, on the "battlefield of the warrior." "Reflective, thoughtful, humble and expectant," Why? It's because God is there.

Remember, God will use everything, even cancer, for the good of those who love him and are called according to his purposes, (*Romans 8:28*). I continue to look for him, waiting on his perfect timing and his impeccable plan for me.

Pastor Dave Bechtel from Bethel Church in Richland, Washington, was the pastor who married Mark and me. He is a remarkably talented teacher of the word of God, so much so, that we continue to listen to his weekly sermons on cassette tapes. He describes his own praying during trial and tribulation this way: "Wow, God! I can't wait to see what you are going to do with *this!*"

My question to you is pretty simple. How different could the process and experience of the cancer diagnosis be, if we could adopt these approaches?

Entry 79

We have been pretty busy after our trip to the American Association of Christian Counselors World Conference in Nashville, Tennessee, as well as a visit with the Willman family in St. Louis. I had every intention of adding to this journal, but the time just slipped away from me and now it's a week after our return.

Two things happened that I want to share. The first is about my childhood friend, Jeanne. The second pertains to a divine appointment arranged at our church.

Jeanne

I have known Jeanne (La Croix) Grant since my elementary school and "Blue-Bird/Camp Fire Girls" days. I remember going over to Jeanne's house to sleep overnight, and staying up into the wee hours of the night talking and listening. Jeanne is *very* passionate. She opens up and shares her life quite easily and gracefully. I mentioned earlier in this journal that she was my try-out partner for cheerleading in Jr. High and High School.

Jeanne and I have reconnected several times over the years, but never at any satisfactory length or depth. The last time I had seen her was at the Richland High "all year" reunion in 2000. Jeanne and her husband, J. Ed, were planning a trip to the Hawaiian Islands a couple years ago, but we never got it together enough to even touch base. This year was different. There was to be a God-ordained purpose for our connecting, and Jeanne did her part by e-mailing me to notify me when she and J. Ed would be coming to Kauai.

Mark and I were off island during the initial days of their stay. I managed to see Jeanne, J. Ed and Jayden, their granddaughter, two times while they were here. It was so good to reconnect with them. Jeanne, in her typical open manner, shared that upon return to Richland, she had scheduled a hysterectomy. She said that there were identified problems that were anticipated to be corrected via surgery. We agreed to pray as they embarked on this journey, not realizing what the Lord had in store for us all.

Jeanne was scheduled for surgery the following Monday, and we left for Tennessee on Tuesday. It was Wednesday when we received a phone call from our "miracle" cat sitter, Luanna. (God used Luanna's willing heart to work a miracle of healing in our precious 14 year old cat, Pumpkin, who is now on her tenth life!) Luanna dutifully relayed the urgent message. It was Jeanne, tearfully letting us know that upon examination prior to her hysterectomy, they discovered cancer. Besides her family, we were the first ones that she called.

As I recall the moment I heard Jeanne's voice on our machine, my eyes watered and I was flooded with emotions.

(There it is, just below the surface of my consciousness; that old familiar pain of hearing the words "You have cancer.")

Next I experienced sadness and dread for what I knew all too well, would be the overwhelming, shocking experience of my dear friend. And finally, there was gratefulness to God for orchestrating our reconnection after so many years... at just the right time, in just the right way. Unbelievable! Unless this was *my* experience, I would seriously consider anyone telling me this story to be exaggerating, stretching the facts to fabricate substantiation of their point. But it *is* my experience. Exaggeration is unnecessary.

I proceeded to return Jeanne's call and we talked for about 45 minutes. Jeanne determined very quickly that the Lord had allowed this event into her life at this time, for the purpose of drawing her back to his side. I assured her that it is my experience that God will go to any length to bring us back into his protective love. At the end of our conversation, Mark joined us on speaker phone from our Tennessee hotel room, and we prayed. Our prayer was deep and heart-felt, with emotional connections that only come from those who have walked the path of the dreaded diagnosis. We heard Jeanne whisper, "not now" and "later honey" several times to her granddaughter who was attempting to attract attention. Our prayer must have gone on over five minutes, and when we finally said, "Amen," Jeanne expressed her thankfulness and surprising relief. At the time, we did not ask for details of her experience. Instead we rested in the peace of knowing that we requested the Lord's healing presence in Jeanne's life, and through our faith and experience, we believed that he would answer our prayer.

Entry 80
Jeanne's Miracle

We had just arrived at sister, Jane Willman's home where we went to celebrate Mark's mother's birthday. My phone rang, noisily announcing its presence with "Hail Purdue," the Purdue University Fight Song. (My cell phone company told me to choose a ring tone that would catch my attention because I was having trouble hearing it. Hail Purdue will always grab my attention!)

I could not locate my phone fast enough to answer it before the darn thing, with irritating efficiency, took a message. I accessed my message and heard Jeanne's voice urging me to get Mark and return her call. I pulled Mark aside, and we went outside to call Jeanne back.

Jeanne spoke to us through her excitement, over-enunciating in an attempt to keep herself from exploding. She described how she had been "telling everyone" about the prayer that Mark and I had prayed over the phone lines just prior to her Seattle surgery trip. She said that during our prayer, she felt as if a huge, comforting "bubble" was forming around her. When we concluded, she sensed an enormous weight flying off her shoulders, and a peace infiltrating her being.

Jeanne continued by telling us that she remained in that peace throughout her surgery process. She expected to receive the test results in a week, dictating the type of chemotherapy she would need. This plan was thwarted after receiving a phone call from her doctor only one day after returning home. The doctor already had such extraordinary, positive results, that he could not wait to share the news with Jeanne and her family! We could hear the tears of joy as Jeanne told us of the doctor's amazement and proclamation of her freedom from chemotherapy.

Jeanne is cancer free. She received a miracle healing from God. She couldn't stop thanking us for our support and love, for sharing our experiences and for demonstrating our faith. We all praised the Lord for his faithfulness, his mercy and his grace. Jeanne said that it was now her turn to encourage another by sharing her story of God's incredible power. (Jeanne had just received a phone call notifying her of someone in her life who had recently been diagnosed with cancer.) We prayed together and hung up the phone with a song in our hearts.

Entry 81
Divine Appointment

The second thing that I wanted to tell you about occurred at our Sunday Church service upon our return from Tennessee. A wonderful brother in the Lord, Mark Beeksma, mentioned to me that there had been a new person attending our church since we had been away. Mark suggested that I connect with this man, because he had expressed an interest in moving to our part of the island. Honestly, I didn't put Mark's suggestion very high on my priority list, but prayed internally that if it was a God appointment, I would be open to it.

During the fellowship time following the sermon, I found myself heading over in the direction of this new church attendee. As I engaged in conversation with Brian Alston, it became clearer to me that God had something for me via this unexpected connection. As we discussed his interests in ecology and island affairs, Brian told me that he additionally teaches education courses on-line, and that he has self-published two books.

OK, God. I hear you. I asked Brian about each of his interests culminating with his advice on self-publication. I had been wondering when the Lord was going to direct me on the next step of this journey. I believe God used this new association as a vehicle for his message to me: finish the book, and then explore publishing options.

Entry 82
You are what owns you

As usual, I was running late to my women's Bible study. I was thinking to myself, "Why is it that no matter what time I get up, I always seem to be late?" Because I am so frequently dealing with this question in my life, I have attempted to focus on what God may have for me on the way to wherever I am going. This day he revealed a treasure to me.

I was listening to our local Christian radio station. A program called "Winning Walk," by Dr. Ed Young, was airing. I do not recall ever hearing this program, but today I believe it was on just for my benefit. Dr. Young said something in his message that I felt compelled to write about:

"The world says you are what you own...God says you are what owns *you!*"

Ed Young was actually talking about money, and the fact that we can let money and possessions influence us to the point that they almost "own" us by consuming our time and directing our lives. But I realized that God wanted me to address this same point from another view. I believe that cancer can own you. It can dictate what you eat, how you sleep, who you see, how you view life, who you relate to, how you feel, what you think, how you spend your time... you get the idea.

I refuse to allow cancer to own me. No matter what happens in my life, cancer will never own me. It is something that happened to me, it did not become me. There is a really neat poem that I received from a wonderful lady at our church named Gladys Uyehara. It also hangs on the office walls of the Kauai American Cancer Society office. It reminds me of the things cancer cannot do:

What Cancer Cannot Do

Cancer is so limited ...
It cannot cripple love,
It cannot shatter hope,
It cannot corrode faith,
It cannot eat away at peace,
It cannot destroy confidence,
It cannot kill friendship,
It cannot shut out memories,
It cannot invade the soul,
it cannot reduce eternal life,
It cannot quench the spirit,
It cannot lessen the power
of the resurrection.
Anonymous

Entry 83
The Jeanne prayer

Today I met with Darlene and discussed how God continues to draw me toward the finish line of this book. After hearing about Jeanne's healing miracle, she made an interesting suggestion.

Dar said, "Val, I just believe that God is going to do miraculous things through this book." Then she stated, "It would definitely add a dimension to the book if you could put Jeanne's prayer into it." She described how Mark and I could outline what we prayed, giving readers a spiritual weapon they could use against cancer. "I love it!" I exclaimed.

I shared the idea with Mark, and he agreed to help me recreate part of our "Jeanne prayer." Together with the Lord's help, we composed a prayer that we believe will be used by God to provide hope, to encourage posturing against cancer, and to foster healing. We urge you to put your name (or your loved one) into the blanks, and *pray*. Gather others to pray with you because there is power in agreement.

Dear Heavenly Father,

We are so grateful to you for hearing our prayers. Thank you for directing us to make all our requests known to you. You are an awesome and living God, and we trust you with all our needs.

By the authority that is bestowed on us as children of God, we bind the spirit of cancer and any weapons that have been formed against _____. We speak directly to this cancer spirit and command you out of _____ body. We render you, spirit of cancer, powerless over the life of _____ and his/her body. Release _____ in the name of Jesus Christ. At the mention of the name of Jesus, every evil spirit must flee. Every knee shall bow and every tongue shall confess that Jesus is Lord of all, and that means Lord of _____. Spirit of cancer you have no jurisdiction over _____. We claim _____ for Kingdom purposes and Kingdom glory. It is his/her right as a son/daughter of God to receive all the benefits and inheritance promised in the word of God. That includes inheriting the right to God's peace, healing and restoration. In Jesus' name we claim these benefits over the life of _____.

We receive your peace to guard all our hearts and our minds. Thank you Lord Jesus.

Amen and Amen (We are all in agreement and *so it shall be!*)

* *This prayer was modeled after* **Philippians 4:6-7, TNIV**, *"Do not be anxious about anything, but in every situation, by prayer and petition, with thanksgiving, present your requests to God. And the peace of God, which transcends all understanding, will guard your hearts and your minds in Christ Jesus."*

Entry 84
A Final Message from God

I believe it is finally time for me to finish this journal. God blessed me with a clear notion of how to do it, during church this past Sunday. Subsequently, I received confirmation via an e-mail from a woman on my "Victory over cancer" list. The reason it was confirming is that I needed to contact this individual prior to writing the final entry, but just hadn't got around to it. In fact, it had been months since I heard even a peep out of this incredible woman of God. I was so grateful to receive verification that she is still alive! (You will understand my relief after you read about her story and the conversation we had.)

I want to first describe something that happened at the 2008 Kauai Women of Faith Conference. The speaker, Debbie Alsdorf from "Design4Living Ministries," presented a message that I believe embodies a vital concept. It is the heart of this journal. In order to drive home the message, Debbie told a story about her dying mother.

Debbie's mother was a believer in Jesus, but for some unknown reason, she faced her death with much fear. Debbie described how she prayed fervently that the Lord would do something to free her mother from the oppression of fear before he took her home to heaven. Although the details elude me, I remember Debbie describing an encounter that her mother had with a spirit she identified as an angel of God. This angel told Debbie's mother not to fear, and also assured her that heaven was real. The angel told her that soon, she would be with the Lord. Debbie went into more specifics of how her mother fearlessly prepared herself for the approaching moment, but what stuck with me from her story was what her mother told Debbie just prior to dying. Her mother said, in reference to the Bible; *"Live as if it were true...because it is."*

And now, please allow me to share my friend's story.

Rebecca Sutter is a remarkable woman of God. I first met her and Pastor Janet Miller, during an effort to create an "Athletic Chaplaincy Program." Madeline Manning Mims, the famous Olympic Track Gold and Silver Medalist, had a heart to develop a ministry for all levels of athletes via a chaplaincy program. Several of us were generously invited to stay with Dr. Thomas Taulbee at his Texas home while we worked to lay the foundation for this project. Thankfully, Pastor Janet and I remained in contact over the succeeding years. When she received my e-mail about my diagnosis and need for prayer, Janet knew who to involve.

Much to my delight, I received the following e-mails from Rebecca. I had no way of knowing about the amazing journey she had taken since our original meeting. It never ceases to amaze me how God orchestrates every detail of our lives, right down to the tuning of our "instruments." Rebecca most certainly has been an instrument of hope and encouragement in so many lives. And now, she would play a breathtakingly beautiful, inspirational tune over my life.

Subject:
Hello, love and MUCH prayer (Rebecca Sutter)
Date: Fri 05/30/08 11:30 AM

Dear Val and Mark:

I just received your e-mail from Janet Miller and love the fact that you are going into this as a victorious warrior fight team. I am the one who loved you immediately at Dr. Tom Taulbee's. With 40 yrs. of advanced medical-surgical and critical care nursing behind me and our loving LORD, I am here to DECLARE that this is beatable. In fact, many times it will make you stronger on the other side. I know that you know not to fear but you know that hoping and coping are more than that. With 366 "fear not's" in the King James Bible, it is a command NOT a request. Also read every healing verse you can always...every day.

Some of what I am writing comes from the fact that since I was with you, I have walked in Heaven. I am also going to send a letter I put out in 2005 to tell of my 12-20-04 home going. I can now walk and talk with portable oxygen and am accepting all He has carried me through knowing that I will live and not die until He wants to keep me. If I can be of any help, call or write.

Your sister and renewed prayer partner,
Rebecca R. Sutter, MN, CNS, D. of Divinity(h)
Nursing Faculty of U. of Texas @ Austin-retired

Subject: Joy and Peace to you-Read (Rebecca Sutter)
Date: Fri 05/30/08 11:47 AM

Here is the letter I mailed out after experiencing a wonderful walk in heaven. I am able to pray for you in a way that others may not be able to. He did say to us to pray "on earth as it is in heaven". So I can, will and have started just a few minutes ago.

Love, Rebecca...fully alive

You too may feel like you have been hit by a truck...I literally was!!!

Hello Everyone!

My husband, Herb and I are glad to be writing to you all. We owe almost every one of you a note of reply but believe you will understand why at the end of this letter. We have appreciated your cards of get well, sympathy, best wishes and Christmas greetings with the pictures and the gifts. In fact, we continue to enjoy them. We are listening to Christmas music as we sign, address and stamp this "long awaited mail out".

Many of you do not know that on October 22, 2002, I was hit from behind and shoved forward into two vehicles. The Jeep left on a flatbed and I left the scene in an ambulance. At the time I was told that all injuries were soft tissue damage. This is a phrase I had used over the years with patients thinking it was a good report of no fractures. Despite all the pain and fatigue, I returned to UT for my students.

Two days later my mother died unexpectedly in Illinois. Upon return from her funeral I closed out the semester while entering physical therapy 3xwk to undo the resultant neck, back, ribs and especially (R) shoulder, arm and hand pain and lack of function.

For almost two years I spent every effort in attempting to leave it all behind. I kept right on working but did not realize what all had happened. I was not able to get pain free and out of serious fatigue. I knew something was wrong but no one had determined what.

Last year on December 18th, I turned in all grades, submitted the required preparatory work for second semester and smiled as I closed my office door at UT that Friday. I was free to enjoy a long break with mission accomplished. I would be going in for "elective" surgery on Monday, returning home that evening with a sling for my (R) shoulder and arm. I believed that I would not need it by the time classes began again in January. I even had every intention to catch up on correspondence, having purchased the cards we are now sending. Oh what a difference a day makes!

One year ago today on December 20th, I died.

When I went in for the surgical repair, the injections were inserted to block the nerves. I knew immediately that I was in trouble. I could not breathe without great effort. It was determined that my phrenic nerve had been shut down as well. This stopped my diaphragm. Next they learned that the left side was out probably from my seat belt injury in the accident and that it had not been working all along. I had been compensating. No wonder I had been declaring my loss of functions and severe fatigue.

We went ahead with heavy respiratory support. I told them to proceed because after two years of pain I could endure anything. "Just fix my shoulder. Keep me awake and stimulated." However, at the end of a very successful repair, I experienced respiratory arrest.

The peace, the love, the music and the beauty of all I visited in heaven is beyond description. I have always believed but now I will not be phased by all the scientific theories of the "dying brain or medications or…". I know it is real myself. There is no room to tell all I saw or heard. What some of my patients have told me is true. There is no doubt.

So I remain on 24hr a day oxygen with what is called BiPap at night. Herb is an excellent caretaker. He has added to the skills he had learned caring for his mother. His skill with oxygen tanks and the kitchen are appreciated. He drives me everywhere. His patience is amazing. When I first came home, I was so weak that I could not even walk ten feet to the bathroom alone. I was not released to go to a pulmonary rehabilitation program until July. I still go 3xwk.

We have lost count of all the appointments with our family doctor, the surgeon, the pulmonary critical care physician and his nurse practitioner and then on to the pulmonary hypertension specialist. These continue. The required examinations of non- and invasive testings are too numerous to describe.

We do not know what we would have done without all the support of the nursing faculty and staff of UT. They have given and given to us. Some have even stayed with Herb through the procedures, driven me to appointments out of town to give Herb a break or after dark if necessarily late. They have showered us with cards, gifts and many meals which they would eat with us for company. Many friends of the community and the Chinese church we had worked with came by for visits, brought surprises and always encouraged us. One by one some of you are finding out and I thank you for your calls now that I am able to take them. The support has been needed and appreciated by both of us. I remain on medical leave from UT.

Slowly I am advancing but am limited due to the fact that my (L) diaphragm remains paralyzed. I have learned to think of myself as a very blessed turtle climbing a mountain path. We have learned much being together every day after years of being gone for long days of service. We have enjoyed laughing, talking and "being".

So how do we close a letter like this one? This truly has been a year of declaring I will live and not die. We know our steps are ordered by the Lord but George Mueller said also the STOPS. I have known Jesus well as the Man of Sorrows but I now covet His name of Shiloh, the Man of Rest. Learning has increased in resting only on God, getting still and waiting before Him until saturated with His presence, then going forward with conscious freshness and "vigor" or as I can. I have truly known to be in the Shadow of His hand, hearing "Sit still, my daughter! Just sit calmly still." I am learning that God never says to "Stand Still, Sit still or Be Still" unless He is going to do something in His set time.

We all claim Peace, Peace be still...do we know great calm? Do we know quietness amid the loss of inward consolations? Are we comforted by the fact that quietness and confidence in God is our joyful strength? It is something else to have to live it.

Spurgeon has said to breathe deeply and I certainly know each breath I take is from God. This Christmas let us learn that in all the hard places God brings us into, He is making opportunities for us to exercise such faith in Him as will bring about blessed results and greatly glorify His name.

I can truly bear witness to the Shekinah Glory of God's Light! Staggering not at the exceedingly great and precious promises, I am certain we can "March on in Strength and Song!" I have been launched out into the very deep. By the God of All Grace, I can shout that I know He can establish, strengthen and settle us. Praise be to God who causes us to triumph and says we ought always to pray and not faint. I have read the Bible and many books, listened to many tapes and movies this year. All that I have taken in declares apparent defeat results in marvelous victory. One quote I love came from Trumbull...those who are readiest to trust God without other evidence than His Word always receive the greatest number of visible evidences of His Love. That's Herb and Rebecca!

Tonight we write to say "God Bless You All". May your joy overflow. The One Who is Unconditional Love is returning.

(Reprinted with permission)

217

Rebecca proceeded to battle on my behalf, literally taking my needs into the heavenly realm. She strengthened me in a "supernatural" manner. When I needed information, she gave that to me. When an encouragement was in order, she offered it up. She invited me to call her, but for several months I put it off. Eventually, Rebecca told me in an e-mail that she wanted me to use the money I might spend to call her, to purchase something for myself. That did it! I knew God was prompting me to call. A couple weeks after the Kauai Women of Faith Conference, I called.

Rebecca answered on the initial ring, and told me that my call was perfectly timed. We reconnected and I asked her to describe her heavenly visit in more detail. For about twenty minutes she portrayed the unfathomable, indescribable depths of color, music, dimensionality and beauty that she encountered in heaven. She continually professed the inadequacy of her vocabulary for communicating such an encounter. As our conversation began to wind down, Rebecca and I were trading scriptures. Suddenly, as if prompted with a shove from behind, she said this:

"Val, you are not reading about my experience in a book, nor are you hearing it second or third hand. You are hearing about it from *me*, your trusted friend and sister in the Lord. I want you to remember something above all else, and that is: *Live as if it were true, because it is!"*

That was my confirmation. In less than two weeks, from two separate sources, God very clearly presented me with a command. And now, at the ending of this "Victory over cancer journey" I want to emphasize the same message to you. With respect to the Living, Breathing, Loving, Merciful, Grace-Filled, All Knowing, Power-Filled God, and His Word, the Bible:

"LIVE AS IF IT WERE TRUE…BECAUSE IT IS!"

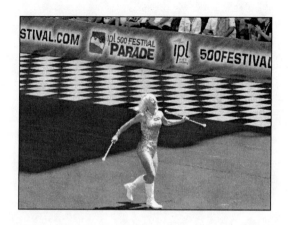

Picture thanks to Scott Sermersheim.

Valerie at the Indianapolis 500 Parade Victory March, twirling on the "carpeted" road past the grandstands

Donations for the ministry, "Victory over cancer: *Live as if it were true…because it is!*" can be made through:

www.drvaleriewillman.com

We encourage you to share with us how God used this publication in your lives. Contact us at:

drval@drvaleriewillman.com or val@jesusanswers.com